Let food be thy medicine
and medicine be thy food.

Hippocrates

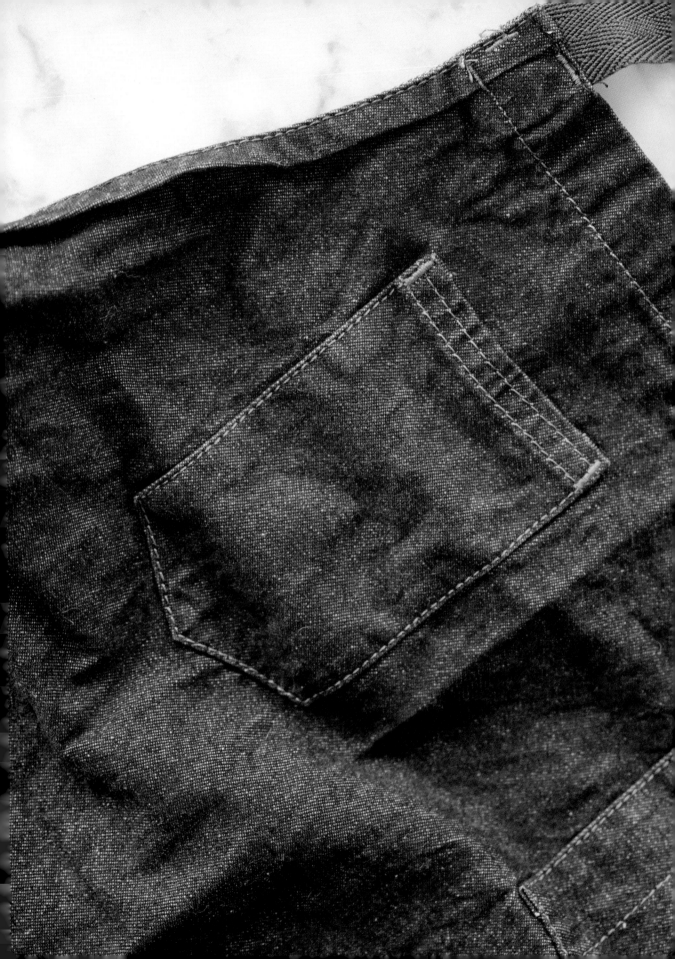

Acknowledgements

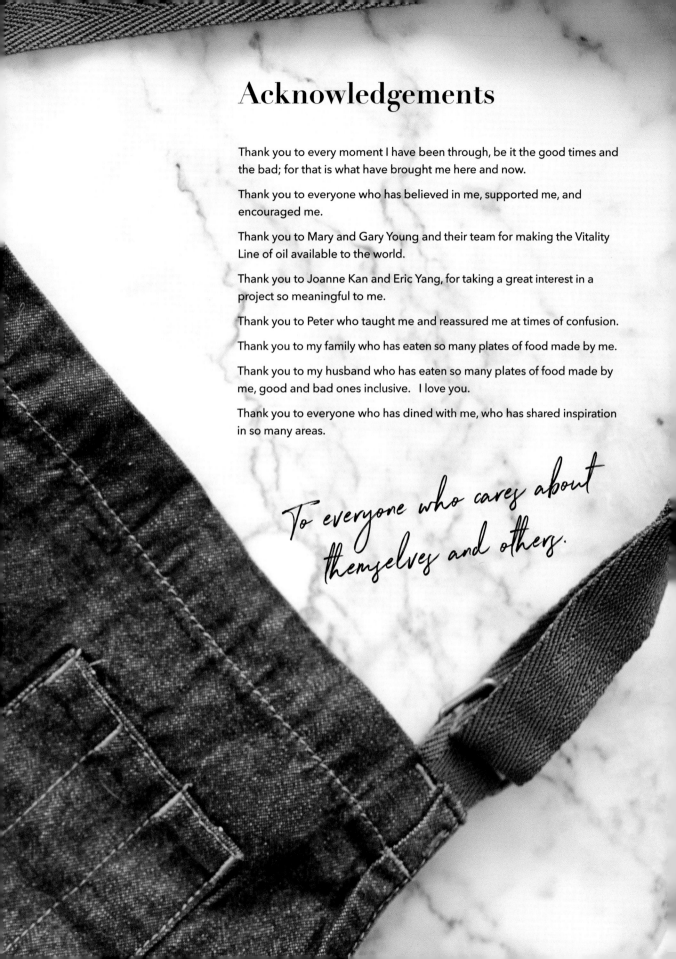

Thank you to every moment I have been through, be it the good times and the bad; for that is what have brought me here and now.

Thank you to everyone who has believed in me, supported me, and encouraged me.

Thank you to Mary and Gary Young and their team for making the Vitality Line of oil available to the world.

Thank you to Joanne Kan and Eric Yang, for taking a great interest in a project so meaningful to me.

Thank you to Peter who taught me and reassured me at times of confusion.

Thank you to my family who has eaten so many plates of food made by me.

Thank you to my husband who has eaten so many plates of food made by me, good and bad ones inclusive. I love you.

Thank you to everyone who has dined with me, who has shared inspiration in so many areas.

To everyone who cares about themselves and others.

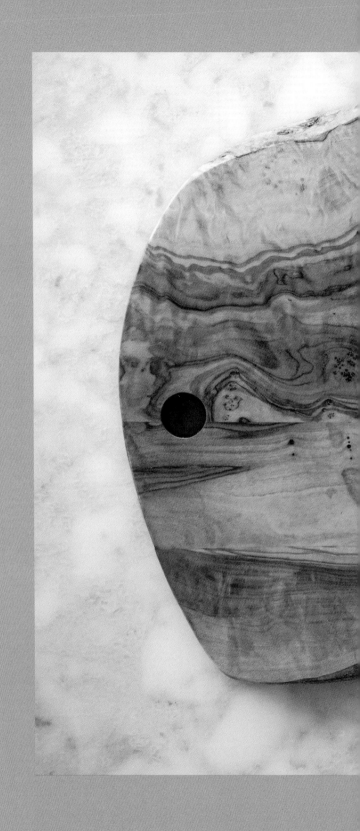

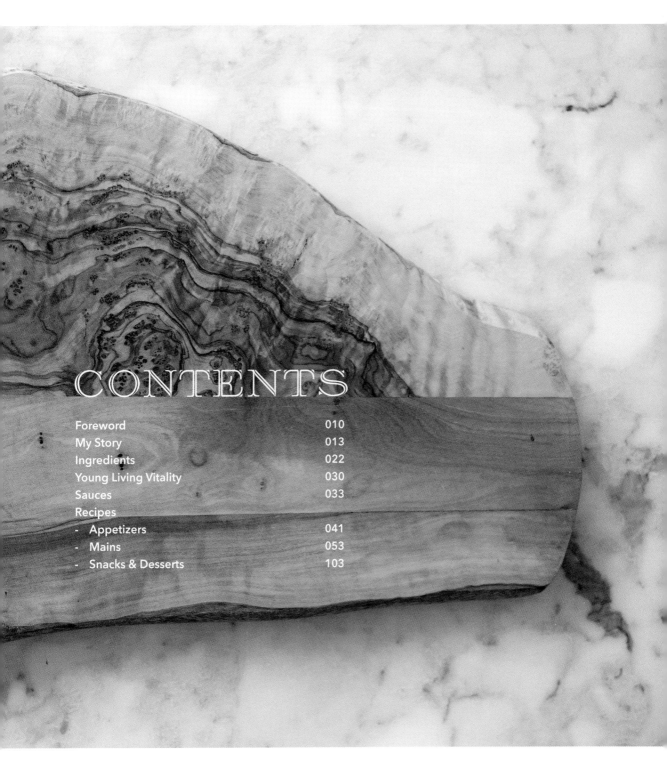

CONTENTS

The power to change the world
for the better is within each of us.

Foreword
by Joanne Kan
Royal Crown Diamond, Young Living Essential Oils

Grace and I were primary school classmates. In school where everyone was competitive, Grace stood out as a soft-spoken, gentle, considerate and kind person. You may have heard her talk at the Biocode Essential Oil Online Symposium 2017 organized by Dr. Olivier Wenke. She was in the Traditional Chinese Medicine (TCM) and Essential Oil talk with me.

Seven years ago, when I told her about these amazing oils she was eager to try. Instead of the Start Living with Everyday Oils, she bought a Basic Start Living Kit, White Angelica, and the Feelings Kit. Later on, she continued to fill her home with Young Living's other products including NingXia® Red. About 2 months into drinking NingXia Red, she thought she had a flu for a very long time. Despite getting treatments from her Chinese doctor and an acupuncturist, she wasn't getting better. That was when she realized she was detoxing. Then she started getting rashes all over. Since then, she's been trying, searching, reading, testing on herself ~ from TCM to energy healing, acupuncture to exercising - Yoga, Pilates, cross training, weights - hypnotherapy to meditation, juicing to diets - vegan, raw food diets, Paleo - whatever she found she was willing to research and try.

Through these years, she has learned and evolved so much. She is my go-to-girl for emotional oil support! When she started incorporating food into her journey, she would send me what she made. Once, she sent me homemade Chocolate truffles with rum and Joy (yes, the oil, and no it's not Vitality!). I popped one in my mouth and soon enough I was laughing. I called her right away and told her the alcohol must have quickly pushed Joy into the blood!! We both laughed. But, Joy isn't a Vitality Oil, so she couldn't officially put it in food.

Fast forward 3 years, last fall, I was sitting in her dining room. She was serving me one of the best gourmet, beautifully cooked, lovingly served Michelin star meals. At Convention two years ago, she started using Light the Fire™, then Live Your Passion™, and after last summer she used Fulfill Your Destiny™ and she just started cooking up a storm (I'm getting goosebumps as I type these words!!). She felt like everything she had learned and done was falling into place.

Just before last Christmas, I invited her to collaborate some of her Vitality recipes to make a little booklet for our team. She told me she hadn't taken any photos nor done anything systematic. She graciously said she would whip up something for me. Two weeks later, she told me she had come up 30 recipes! (Her exact words were, "I downloaded 30 recipes.") A few weeks later she was sending me photographs of beautifully cooked food, and mouthwatering recipes. I looked through what she had sent me and I said to myself, "These are too good not to share with the world. I cannot just keep them for my own team's use."

I connected with Troie Storms-Battles, CEO and Partner of Life Science Publishing, and showed her Grace's work. She was as excited, as we were! Grace does not expect this to become a top seller or to make a lot of money. This book is to show you that you can easily use the amazing Vitality Line + kitchen staple food to whip up something that is easy, delicious and healthy. After all, as Grace says, we all have to eat three meals a day. And as cliche as it is, we ARE what we eat.

While you are looking and trying out the recipes, please also read the excerpts written by Grace. You'll get a glimpse of my beautiful friend. Grace also makes her own pet food. I hope that her next work is a little booklet for home-made pet foods.

Grace lives in Hong Kong with her husband, little Sean (Bichon Frise), the happiest Young Living doggy I've met, and the new addition to her family Tang Tang.

MY STORY

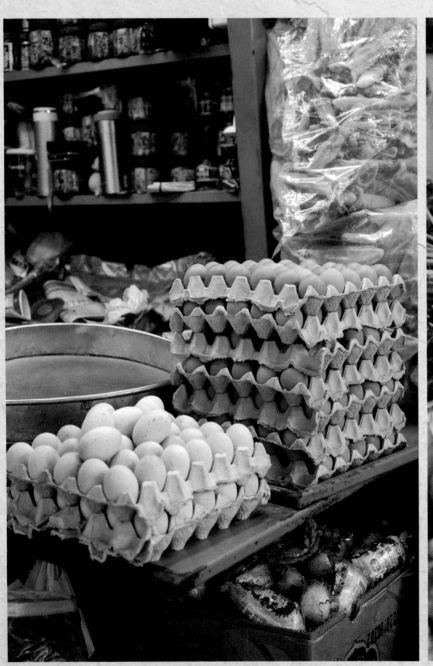
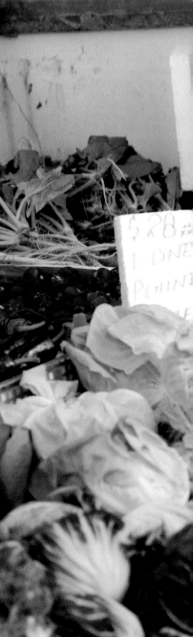

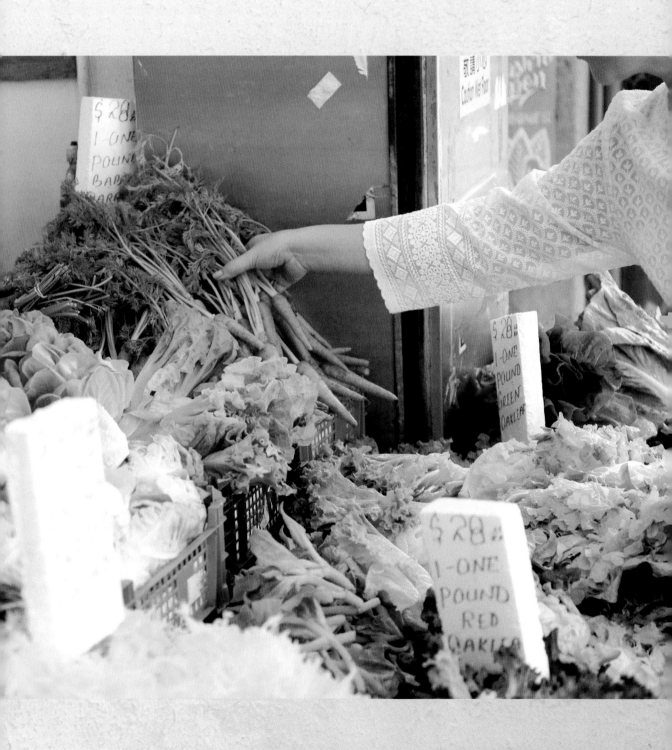

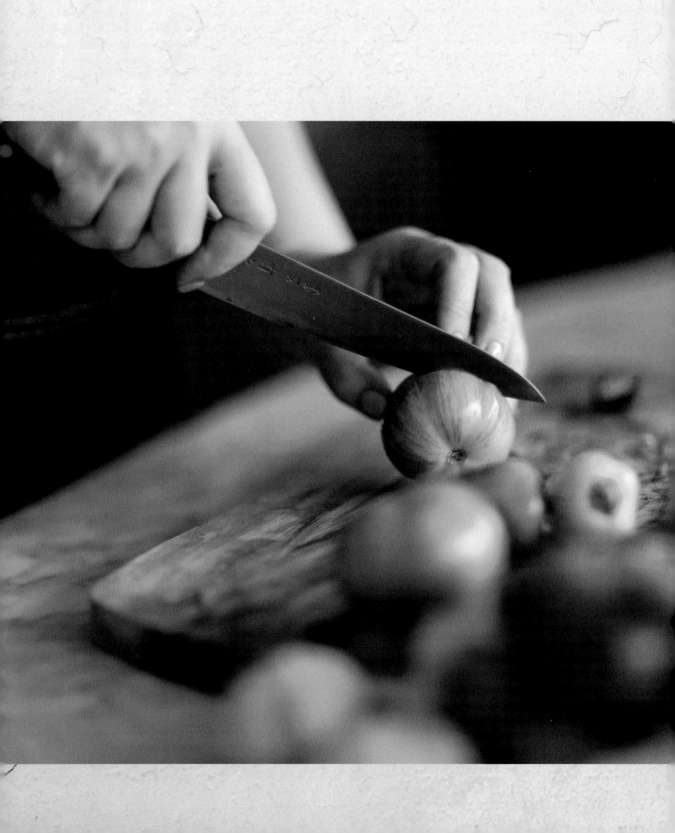

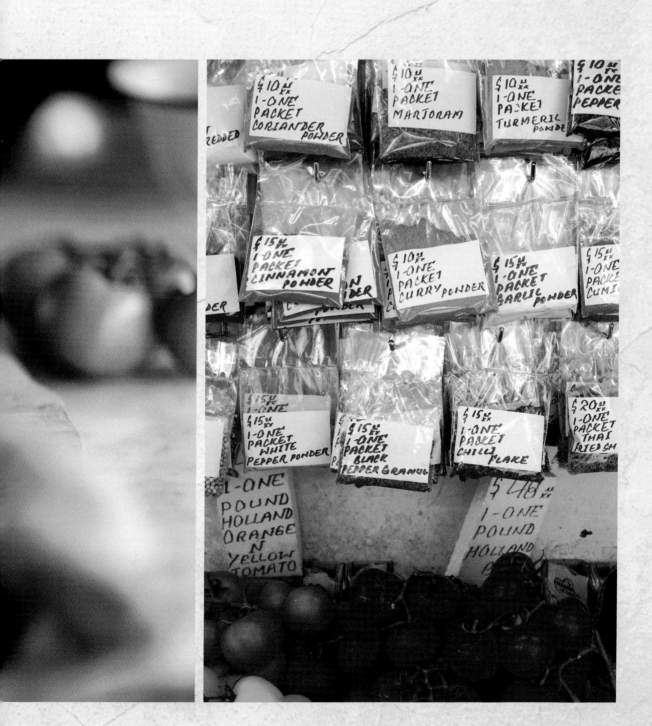

ABOUT
·
GRACE

Grace Lee, an ardent cook, views cooking as a cathartic process. For her, cooking a meal for family and friends can assist in purging emotional tensions and stress, and bring a sense of balance and well-being after a tough day. She has spent many years establishing an intimate relationship with tools, ingredients and cooking methodologies, some of which are rooted in ancient Chinese traditions that she picked up from the elders in her family. Her cuisine has an amalgamation of Asian and Western flavors, some of which she picked up from her time in San Francisco. Only the freshest of ingredients are allowed in her kitchen, to create little plates of art that rouse the senses. No matter what culture one belongs to, food is the common thread that has the power to bring people together and this is what she aspires toward.

Grace's passion for cooking has its seeds in a difficult journey. In her mid-30s she suffered a mini stroke which was a serious wake up call for her. For over a decade she underwent numerous alternative treatments; TCM, Tibetan medicine, Qi Gong, acupuncture, different holistic remedies, gym, yoga, meditation and Young Living Essential Oils. After having tried numerous diets; Atkins, paleo, keto, raw, vegetarian, vegan, pescatarian she concluded that there is no need to limit the ingredients she uses in her cooking, instead striking a balance with everything wholesome. Her love of home-made

sauces, fermented foods and essential oils from **Young Living's Vitality Series** is evident in her dishes. The goal for her is to always create unique rich flavors that arouse one's senses and linger on one's palate. She realized that good health is a blessing that must be nurtured through a balanced heart, body and mind. This is when cooking became a form of meditation for Grace. She found herself so calm, still and centered throughout the cooking process, the energy felt divine and she found herself spending more and more time preparing meals for her family and friends.

Grace's perspective on food procurement, preparation and consumption is grounded in the reverence for our planet. "Our planet is our home; our bodies are our temples and it is crucial to act conscientiously. You wouldn't harm your home or place of worship, would you?" Her cooking philosophy is to bring mindfulness and awareness back to everyday consumption of food. She is a strong proponent of intuitive eating that allows us to respect not just our bodies, but also our planet. Intuitive eating speaks with our body, mind and soul; it reminds us to slow down, listen, and pay attention to the messages and signs that our bodies and nature gives us. These messages could include hunger, cravings, addictions, allergies, mood swings, shifts in energy levels, discomfort, and pleasure. She believes that by paying attention to

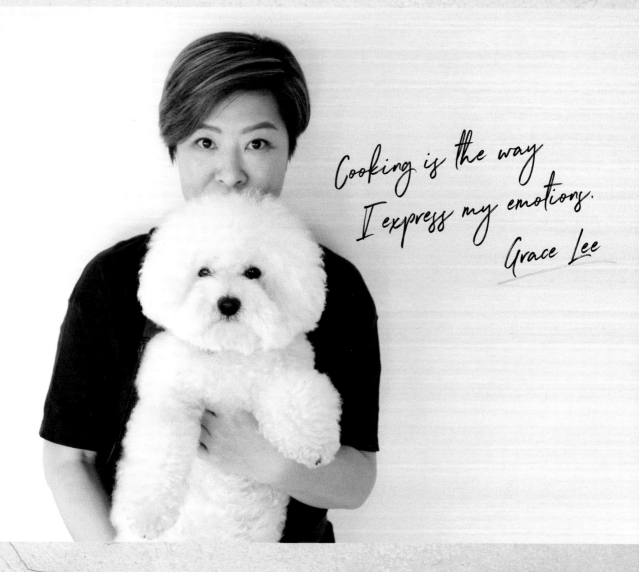

Cooking is the way
I express my emotions.
Grace Lee

the signals that our bodies give us, we can train and alter our visual, auditory, gustatory, olfactory and tactile senses and embrace meditative cooking and mindful eating.

Through her cooking, Grace is determined to help people become more aware of their senses and their bodies. She wishes to ignite an interest in people; for fresh, wholesome, organic foods, buying locally produced foods, eating more fruits and vegetables, consuming fewer packaged products, preparing sauces and entire meals from scratch, using natural seasonings and supporting companies that are dedicated to protecting the environment and giving back to society. According

to Grace, this is the only way that we can positively impact our health, wealth and environment.

She reminds readers, "Have fun and be creative with recipes, don't restrict yourself. Play with the ingredients, substitute them; use soy sauce instead of tamari or coconut sugar instead of agave. Always remember food culture is all about sharing a piece of your heart with the people you love and with strangers to build relationships and memories, but more importantly to celebrate life and love. We must never forget that love is the most essential ingredient."

The secret ingredient
is always love

Ingredients

What we put in our bodies is the foundation of our overall healthy.

That's why I cook with wholesome ingredients whenever I can. That translates to ingredients that your body appreciates. That also translate to foods that you see in their real form. A broccoli is a kind of wholesome food, a slice of chicken thigh is also wholesome. But, a can of broccoli cream soup or a chicken nugget isn't what I'd call wholesome. Every decade or so, there is a hype on a certain type of food in the market. Superfood is what everyone is talking about now; whereas milk and dairy was the hype back then in the 90s. Judge for yourself what works and what doesn't. Listen to your body; observe how your body reacts after eating a certain type of food. Remember your body is your best friend. What works for others, might not necessarily work for you. Some like wheat, others don't. Gluten free might work for some, but doesn't work for everyone.

I try to strike a balance on what I eat. There are days when I have consumed too much deep fried or grilled meats, and I will end up feeling heaty. I sometimes get a headache and feel more agitated than normal, perhaps because of too much heat in the liver. I then adjust my diet and go for green smoothies for the following mornings or simply add a drop of Peppermint Vitality™ to my teas. Nature is very smart and there is always a solution to a problem; it is just up to our awareness.

I live in Hong Kong and am very lucky to get a wide variety of ingredients. I go for local ingredients when I can, other times I go for foods that are vacuumed sealed and flash-frozen too. Foods packed this way capture the peak of freshness, it also ensures a very high level of nutrient density, flavor and protein. Many of the recipes here involve Asian ingredients. Most of these ingredients can be found in Asian

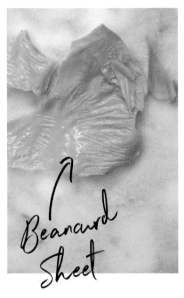

Beancurd Sheet

supermarkets. I have made a brief listing here to help better understand what they are and why they make good ingredients our bodies will appreciate.

I also use sweets and seasonings that provide a healthier or gluten free option. If you already have these in your kitchen, that's great. If not, try them next time you get to a health food store.

Agave is a sweetener derived from agave sap, it has very low GI, low in glucose and doesn't spike blood.

Arrowroot Flour (葛粉) is an excellent thickening agent used in making sauces and stews. It is extracted from the Marantaceae family of plants and is nutritionally dense. I like to use this in place of cornstarch that is often called for in Chinese cooking.

Coconut Aminos is an alternative to soy sauce. It is made from raw coconut tree sap that's aged naturally. It is gluten free, soy free and has much lower sodium compared with soy sauce. It contains 17 amino acids and vitamin B and C plus other minerals.

Balacan Malaysian Prawn Paste (馬拉盞) is one of the most commonly used ingredients in Malaysian cooking. It is a hardened block of shrimp paste made from tiny shrimp that's fermented. It adds depth to cooking and is less oily when compared to say Thai shrimp paste.

Beancurd Sheet (腐竹) is a tofu sheet made from soybeans. There are chilled ones and dried ones. If using the dried ones, make sure you soak them in water first in order to rehydrate.

Canned Abalone can be found in better Asian Grocery Stores or places where they sell dried herbs and dried seafood. Abalone is considered a delicacy in Asian ingredients. Fresh abalone is favored by chefs, however if you're a home cook and don't have the access to fresh ones, the canned ones are very convenient to use. On the top or the bottom of the can where there are numbers printed, it shows the number of pieces of abalone per can.

Chili Oil gives an ambient heat to food. There are store bought ones readily available that are made with soy oil. Chili Oil should be clear and reddish in color. If you want to make your own, simply cook oil until it is very hot (190C). Then pour oil over a combination of chili flakes, star anise and let it infuse. Just make sure you use a ceramic bowl or heat proof glass jar. And take care and not to burn yourself.

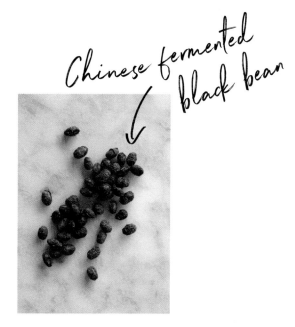

Chinese fermented black bean

Chinese Celery is also called leaf celery. It is a variety of celery grown in East Asian countries. The fragrant is more pungent and peppery when compared to western celery.

Chinese Fermented Black Bean (黑豆豉) is widely used to make black bean sauce or black bean paste. You can buy these semi dried from Asian grocery stores. Although they call this a black bean, these are actually soy beans. It is during the fermentation that has made the soy beans black in color.

Chinese Sweet Bean Paste (甜面醬) is a thick, opaque, smooth, dark brown paste with a mild savory sweet flavor. The sauce is made primarily from fermented flour, along with salt. This is not a wheat free ingredient.

Chinese Rose Wine (玫瑰露酒) is a cooking wine made from sorghum wine and distilled rose petals, sugar and salt. It has an alcohol content of 46% and up.

Coconut Sugar is a natural sweetener I find a lot more flavorful than granulated white sugar. For this reason, I find myself needing less amount of sugar when compared to when using granulated sugars. It also hold trace amount of vitamins and minerals.

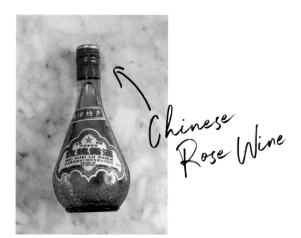

Chinese Rose Wine

Light and Dark Soy Sauce are the two most commonly used seasonings used in Chinese cooking. These two are very similar except the dark soy sauce is aged for a longer period of time and with molasses or caramel. It is also thicker in color and more full-bodied flavored. It is less salty and can be used to create an almost sweet and savory taste. Soy sauce is made with fermented wheat and is mostly non-gluten free. Soy sauce is rich in antioxidants, isoflavones and protein, with traces of vitamin B6. Look for brands that use non GMO crops when using soy sauce.

Dulse Flakes is referred to as a sea vegetable or marine algae. It is low in fat but high in protein and vitamins. There is a natural saltiness in flavor in dulse and can be eaten as snacks or used as a thickening agent or adding more depth in flavor when used in cooking.

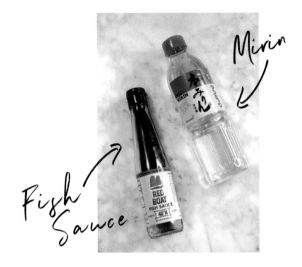

Mirin

Fish Sauce

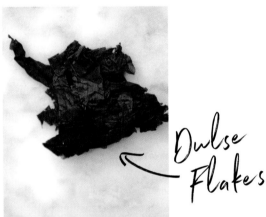

Dulse Flakes

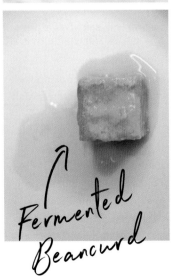

Fermented Beancurd

Fermented Beancurd (腐乳) is a salty condiment in that is made by preserving tofu with salt, rice wine and sesame oil. There are different types of it such as white fermented tofu and red fermented tofu. It has a soft and spreadable texture and is often referred to as Chinese Cheese.

Sweet Fermented Rice (酒釀) is made with glutinous rice that is fermented with distiller's yeast. It is often used in making desserts. According to traditional Chinese cooking wisdom, sweet fermented rice has ability to 'warm your insides' and improve blood flow. With updated research; it turns out sweet fermented rice may have similar health benefits such as yogurt, only this is dairy-free!

Fish Sauce is a condiment made from fermenting fish with salt. It has a rich translucent reddish brown color and adds a savory complexity to dishes. There are a couple gluten free brands out there that yield beautiful results too.

Gojujang is a Korean red chili paste that is savory sweet and spicy fermented condiment that is made from chili powder, glutinous rice, fermented soybean, barley malt powder and salt. It is one of the most commonly used Korean condiments.

Ghee is a type of clarified butter that is full of fat-soluble vitamins and healthy fatty acids. Ghee has a high smoke point and is an excellent option to cooking oil. Some studies suggest that ghee has many health benefits too. Look for grass fed ghee options.

Maple Sugar is a delicious healthier sweetener alternative made entirely of maple syrup. It has a very gentle and mild sweetness and has a higher level of nutrients, antioxidants and phytochemicals than granulated white sugar. Sugar is sugar though, consume moderately.

Mirin (味醂) is a Japanese sweet rice wine that gives a sweet tangy flavor. It is similar to sake but has a lower alcohol content and higher sugar content. The sugar is a complex carbohydrate that forms naturally during the fermentation process, so no added sugar is needed.

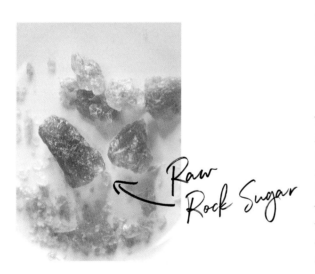

Raw Rock Sugar

Raw Rock Sugar (冰糖) is made from unrefined sugar with a rich aroma. Traces of mineral can be found in raw rock sugar. It is a healthier choice and often used in Chinese braising.

Rice Flour (粘米粉) is a staple food in Asian cooking. It is a form of flour made from finely milled rice. It is a good substitute for wheat flour and sometimes used as a thickening agent.

Rice Noodle is often found sold dried in various widths. It is made with milled rice and is gluten free. Substitute this for noodles or pastas. The most common rice noodles are found in white color, but you can also find them in various colors such as black or brown depending on the type of rice used.

Tamari is an alternative to soy sauce. It is made with mostly soybeans and no wheat nor other grains. Look for MSG-free options and brands that use non-GMO crops.

Tapioca Starch (木薯粉) is made from the root of cassava plant. It is gluten free, wheat free and is neutral in taste. When used as a starch coating for deep fries, tapioca starch gives a thicker and translucent 'crust' which picks up more sauce and gives more mouth-feel.

Tahini is a condiment made from ground sesame seeds. Commercial tahini is usually made from white, hulled sesame seeds. You can make your own too where you can decide if you want raw, sprouted, toasted or sesame seeds. Tahini has a high fat content, adds texture and helps bind ingredients together.

Taro Root is an edible corm from the family of Araceae plants. The part we eat is the root that's mostly underground stem where the nutrients are stored. Taro can be boiled, steamed or oven-baked. Cook thoroughly to prevent mouth and throat itchiness. Also when cutting taro, you might want to wear a glove or use a cloth to prevent direct contact as you might find an itchiness sensation after touching a taro root.

Potato Starch is a starch extracted from potatoes. Similar to arrowroot or tapioca starch this makes a good thickening agent for sauces and coating for deep fries.

Oyster Sauce is a thick, brown sauce with a sweet, savory and earthy flavor. It is full of umami and gives recipes an extra oomph. Look for premium brands for the real oyster umami flavor. (Unless if you're crazy enough like me who makes my own - look for recipes online! It's easier than you think.)

Satay Paste is commonly used in Malaysian cooking. There are a lot of commercial brands to choose from. Opt for the ones with less msg and chemicals. Alternatively, you can very easily make you own too, blending together equal amounts of Thai red curry paste and peanut butter plus coconut sugar to taste.

Sesame Oil is an edible vegetable oil derived from sesame seeds. It has an aromatic and nutty aroma. The oil is nutrient rich and is popular in alternative medicine from traditional massages and treatments.

Seaweed Flakes (Furikake) is a dry Japanese seasoning used for sprinkling on rice. Furikake comes in a wide variety of flavors, from vegan options to variations with dried eggs.

Nori Sheets are red algae that are most commonly used as the wrap of sushi. These can be easily bought in Japanese grocery stores.

Spring Onion is very similar to scallion. Fresh spring onion should have firm and unblemished bulbs with green perky leaves. Both can be used interchangeably.

Shallot is a close relatives of garlic, leek and chive... It is copper, reddish in color and looks like a small onion but has a milder and sweeter taste of an onion with hints of garlic.

Sichuan Peppercorn is a tiny reddish brown peppercorn that is strong and pungent in flavor. The main difference between this and other peppercorns is its interesting mouth-numbing spice. It can be paired with chili peppers or other peppercorns.

Shaoxing Wine is a Chinese wine fermented from rice used for drinking and cooking. Shaoxing is a region in China. If you can't find Shaoxing wine, use dry sherry as a substitute.

Shiso Leaf is in the mint family and is used extensively in Japanese cuisine. It is sometimes called perilla or sesame leaf. It has a distinct, refreshing taste that's quite irresistable. If you can't find them in your Japanese grocery stores, try to find alternatives such as peppermint leaves, basil or rocket salad leaves instead.

Shishito Pepper is from the capsicum family. It has a distinctive flavor with some sweetness and a hint of smokiness. Slender in shape and bright green in color, it is beautiful and elegant on its own.

Shimeji Mushroom is rich in umami tasting and is an edible mushroom that's native to East Asia. Like most mushrooms, it has a woody flavor. Once seasoning is added, the flavor becomes complex and multilayered.

Shitake Mushroom is an edible mushroom that's native to East Asia. It is the second most popular mushroom in East Asia and is considered a medicinal mushroom in some forms of TCM.

Water Chestnut isn't a nut but an aquatic vegetable. It is a low-calorie vegetable that contains no cholesterol and fat. It has a crunchy texture and contains potassium, copper and manganese.

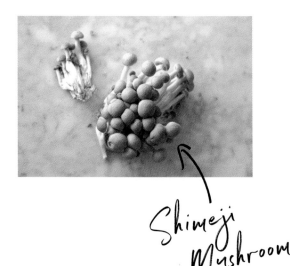

Shimeji Mushroom

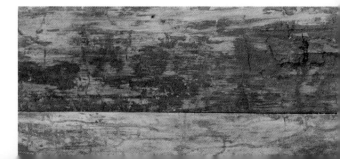

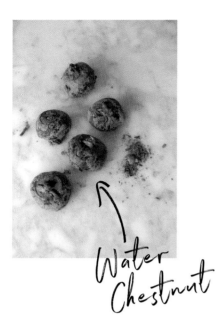

Water Chestnut

Wood Ear Fungus ranges from gray-brown to black in color, rubbery in texture. It resembles the shape of an ear and grows in wood. These are commonly sold in Asian markets dried. Simply soak in water again to rehydrate them for use. Wood Ear Fungus is low in calories and high in protein, iron, vitamin B and dietary fiber.

Japanese White Miso is made from soybeans that have been fermented with a large percentage of rice. This can be found in Japanese markets. The color ranges from light yellow to beige. It has a distinct taste with mild sweetness and creates umami in cooking. There is a lot of sodium in the fermented miso, so do adjust the amount of salt used when cooking with this ingredient.

White Turnip looks like an oversized radish or a white carrot. Unlike peppery radishes, white turnips have a delicate sweet flavor. Choose the ones that are heavy in weight, these tend to be more tender and juicy.

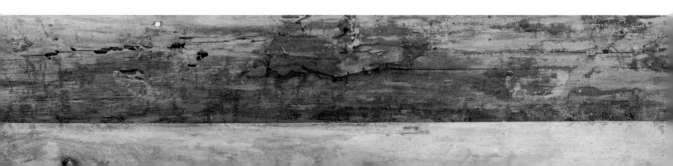

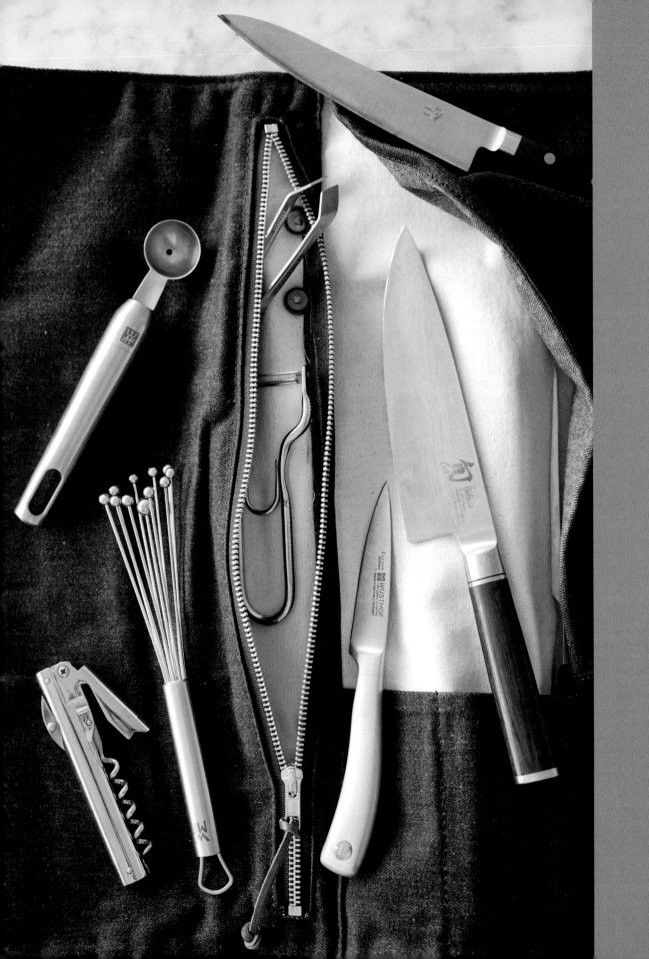

Measurements

Most measurements in this book are shown in American units, such as teaspoonful, tablespoonful, ounce or by the cup. There are times when I have the leisure to spend half a day preparing for a meal, but most of the time I need to make it quick and make it good. The idea behind the way I measure the ingredients is to keep every step convenient and easy to manage in the kitchen. When in doubt, use 'common sense' and have 'fun.' In the kitchen, there's no such thing as right or wrong!

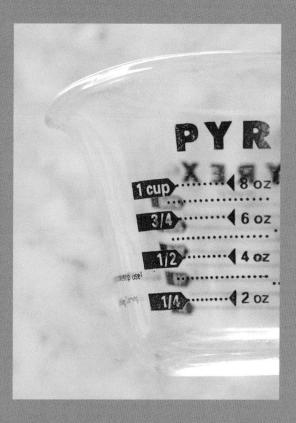

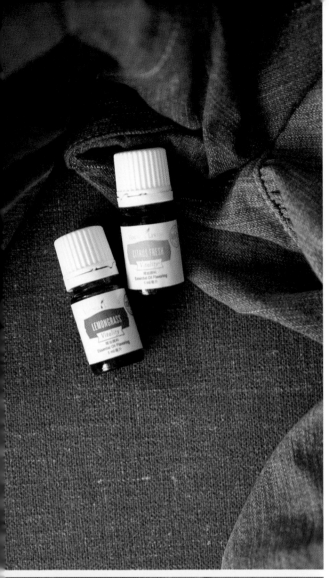

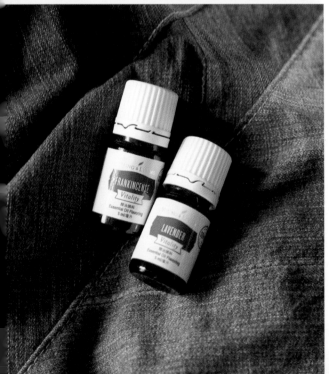

Young Living Vitality Oil

I have to be honest; and, yes I'm a fan of Young Living. Since the launch of the vitality line, I have gotten super excited. Why? Because it's too convenient! The little bottles have contents that are packed with flavors, they're non-GMO & FDA approved! It's pure plant product with nothing else! I could go on, but you get the idea. What's more convenient than simply adding a drop of Ginger Vitality™ to a pork marinade instead of chopping and juicing a stack of ginger slices? And for those who have tried making your own black pepper sauce, you'll be very pleased to know that a couple drops of Black Pepper Vitality™ will take care of your entire batch of sauce.

Cooking with essential oils is easy. Just remember, oils are very concentrated; start with less, you can always add more. Don't let the essential oil overwhelm your dish. Getting the right flavors is all about balancing. If you aren't certain about just getting that one drop from the bottle, use a spoon and drop the oil onto the spoon first before you stir it in your food. There are times when I describe the amount of vitality oil used as a 'hint.' This is when I use a toothpick to touch the orifice of the essential oil bottle. Try this: pick up a bottle of essential oil and tilt the bottle to one side until you see oil collecting on the orifice. Touch a toothpick in the oil for two seconds, then swirl the toothpick in your food. Voila!!

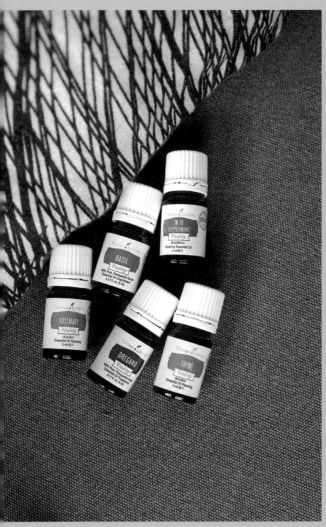

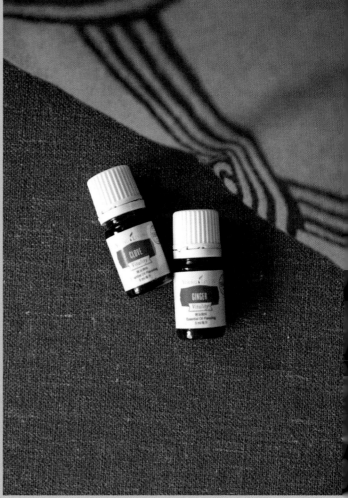

SAUCES

When I was a child, rice was a staple food in my daily diet. I have always loved rice because it goes with everything. My favorite was to eat the plain rice with a sunny-side-up egg that was fried until the edge was slightly burned and crispy, the white remained fluffy while the yolk remained oozy. To make that even more extraordinary, I ladled over a tablespoon of rendered pork fat seasoned with soy sauce, then topped it with some pork rind. That is probably still one of my favorite comfort foods; and THAT is the magic of a sauce. It elevates the flavor and texture of everything.

Sauces can be ladled over pasta or rice, stirred into soup or slathered on a chunk of meat or fish. It can also make cooking at home quicker than you could imagine because sauces can be made ahead of time. For most of the sauces in this cookbook, they can be prepared ahead of time and stay good for a week or so if kept in airtight jars and stored in the refrigerator.

The portion for each of the sauce recipes is small and makes just enough for one or two dishes. You can double or triple the recipe; but I do not recommend sizing it down. A blender is ideal when it comes to making sauces, but a good food processor will do the job too.

There are 12 sauce recipes in this book, but the number of dishes you can create with them can be endless. The recipes I have provided can be your inspiration; do have fun and create your own or adapt them in your favorite dishes.

Basil Spinach Pesto

Goes well as dip, sandwich spread, pasta, on minestrone or grilled meats.

Ingredients

Toasted Walnuts or Pinenuts	½ cup
Salad Spinach Leaves	3 cups
Anchovies	4
(or Balacan Malaysian Prawn Paste 1 tsp)	
Garlic	2 cloves
Lemon Juice	1 tbsp
Olive oil	3 tbsp
Lemon Vitality™	1 drop
Basil Vitality™	hint
Salt	½ tsp
Agave	½ tsp
Fresh Ground Black Pepper	½ tsp

Method

1. Put spinach, nuts, garlic, anchovies /prawn paste, garlic, and lemon juice in a blender.

2. Blend until coarsely chopped.

3. Combine olive oil with Lemon Vitality and Basil Vitality, and add in the blender.

4. Blend until well combined.

5. Season with salt and pepper to taste.

Chinese Recipe p.120

Black Pepper Sauce

Goes well with beef and chicken.

Ingredients

Shallots, finely chopped	8 or Yellow Onion x ½
Garlic, minced	4 cloves
Butter	1 tbsp
Arrowroot Flour	2 tbsp
Agave	1 tsp
Sugar	1 tsp
Stock	13 oz
Dark Soy Sauce	½ tsp
Oyster Sauce	1 tsp
Black Pepper Vitality™	4 drops
Fresh Ground Pepper	¼ tsp
Salt	to taste

Method

1. In a pan, melt butter with low heat; sweat garlic and onion until it's translucent. Take care not to use high heat as you don't want to burn the ingredients.

2. Add the teaspoonful of fresh ground pepper and sauté until it's fragrant.

3. Add in the flour and stir with a spoon to form a roux.

4. Slowly stream in the stock and whisk down to form a sauce.

5. As the sauce thickens, add in the agave and salt to taste.

6. Turn heat off and add in the Black Pepper Vitality.

Chinese Recipe p.120

Essential Oil Infused Balsamic Glaze

Goes well with chicken, duck breast, tomato salad, strawberries, ice cream.

Ingredients

Balsamic Vinegar	⅓ cup
Your choice of Vitality	1 drop
Agave	1 tsp
Black Pepper	
(optional, leave this out if you're using this recipe for desserts)	
Sesame Oil	2 drops
(optional, leave this out if you're using this recipe for desserts)	

Method

1. In a small pot, simmer balsamic vinegar and reduce to ¼ of its volume. About 6-7 minutes, depending on your vinegar. Note that when the vinegar cools, it will thicken up.

2. Add agave, Grapefruit Vitality™ and black pepper to taste.

Other suggestions:

Chinese Recipe p.120

Gochujang Citrus Fresh Dressing

Goes well with seafood and meats. Can be used as dipping sauce, condiment or marinade.

Ingredients

Gochujang	2 tbsp
Citrus Fresh Vitality™	6 drops
Agave	2 tbsp
Fish Sauce	3 drops
Rice Vinegar	2 tbsp
Olive Oil	1 tbsp
Garlic, minced	1 clove
Tamari	1 tsp

Method

1. Whisk together all ingredients until well combined.

Chinese Recipe p.120

Jade Lemon with Fermented Beancurd Sauce

Goes well with lamb.

Can be used as a dressing for salad in place of blue cheese dressing.

Ingredients

Fermented Beancurd	4 squares
Jade Lemon Vitality™	2 drops
Agave	1 tbsp
Sesame Oil	4 drops
Olive Oil	1 tbsp

Method

1. In a bowl, mix together fermented beancurd cubes with Jade Lemon Vitality.

2. Add agave to taste.

3. Add sesame oil and olive oil to achieve desired consistency.

Lemon Lime Spicy Sauce

Goes well with abalone, steamed fish, grilled pork.

Ingredients

Bird's Eye Chili	1
Garlic	2 cloves
Parsley	1 tbsp
Lemon Vitality™	1 drop
Lime Vitality™	1 drop
Water	2 tbsp
Fish Sauce	2 tbsp
Agave	1 tbsp

Method

1. Mince chili, garlic, and parsley and place them in a jar.

2. Add to the jar the rest of the ingredients and shake well.

Lemon Balsamic Tahini with Red Chili Oil

Goes well with cold noodles, cucumber salad, chicken salad, wonton.

Ingredients

Chili Oil	1 tbsp
Olive Oil	1 tbsp
Spring Onion	1 tsp
Minced Garlic	1 clove
Balsamic Vinegar	1 tbsp
Tamari	¼ tsp
Tahini / Peanut Butter	1 tbsp
Agave	1 tsp
Lemon Vitality™ / Lime Vitality™	3 drops

Method

1. Mix all ingredients together well until combined.

Chinese Recipe p.121

Peanut Dipping Sauce

Ingredients

Peanut Butter	1 tbsp
Tamari	1 tsp
Agave	1 tsp
Citrus Fresh Gojujang Sauce (p.035)	¼ tsp
Fresh Lime Juice	½ lime

Method

1. Mix all ingredients together well until combined.

Chinese Recipe p.121

Rosemary Black Bean Sauce

Goes well with pasta, noodles (Jajang Mien), clams, mussels

Ingredients

Olive Oil	2 tbsp
Chinese Fermented Black Bean	2 tbsp
Rosemary Vitality™	a touch
Ginger, minced	1 slice
Garlic, minced	1 clove
Shallots, sliced	2 cloves
Chili, chopped	1
White Pepper	¼ tsp
Agave	1 tsp
Tamari	1 tsp
Squid Ink	2 tsp

Method

1. Mix all ingredients together until well combined.

Soy Jade Lemon Butter Sauce

Goes well with seafood and meats.

Ingredients

Butter or ghee	1 tbsp
Shallots, sliced	1 clove
Apple Cider Vinegar	1 ½ tbsp
Chicken Stock	3 tbsp
Tamari or Soy Sauce	2 tbsp
Mirin	1 tbsp
Jade Lemon Vitality™	3 drops

Method

1. In a small pot, heat the butter. Add shallots to sweat until fragrant, take care not to brown.

2. Add vinegar, chicken stock and tamari; bring to a simmer. Reduce the liquid by half. About 2-3 minutes.

3. Switch off the heat and add in the Jade Lemon Vitality.

Tangerine Thyme Sticky Sauce

Goes well with chicken and prawns.

Ingredients

Garlic, minced	2 cloves
Chili, chopped	2
(deseed them to make a less spicy version)	
Minced Ginger	1 tsp
Tangerine Vitality™	3 drops
Thyme Vitality™	1 drop
Ginger Vitality™	touch
Sugar	1 ½ tbsp
Rice Vinegar	½ tbsp
Soy Sauce / Tamari	2 ½ tbsp
Sesame Oil	2 tsp

Method

1. Add everything except the essential oils to a pan.

2. By using low heat, melt the sugar and combine the ingredients to make a sauce.

3. Turn heat off. Add Tangerine Vitality, Thyme Vitality and Ginger Vitality.

Chinese Recipe p.122

Wasabi Citrus Fresh Salsa Verde

Goes well with grilled fish and other grilled white meats.

Ingredients

Wasabi paste	¾ tsp
Olive oil	2 ½ oz
Parsley	⅓ oz
Rocket Leaves	¼ oz
Capers, very well rinsed	2 tbsp
Fish Sauce	½ tbsp
Garlic, minced	1 clove
Citrus Fresh Vitality™	2 drops
Lemon Vitality™	2 drops
Water	

Method

1. Put wasabi in a small bowl. Slowly stream in the olive oil with one hand, while whisking it in with the other hand.

2. Transfer the wasabi paste mixture to a blender and add the rest of the ingredients to it.

3. Blitz in a food processor to form a coarse puree.

Chinese Recipe p.122

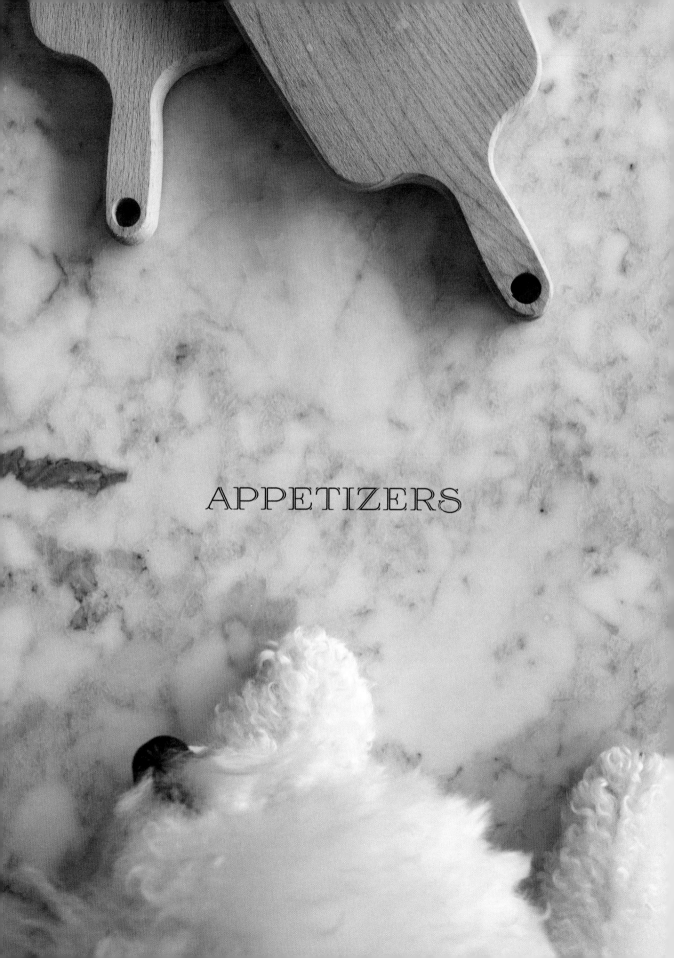

APPETIZERS

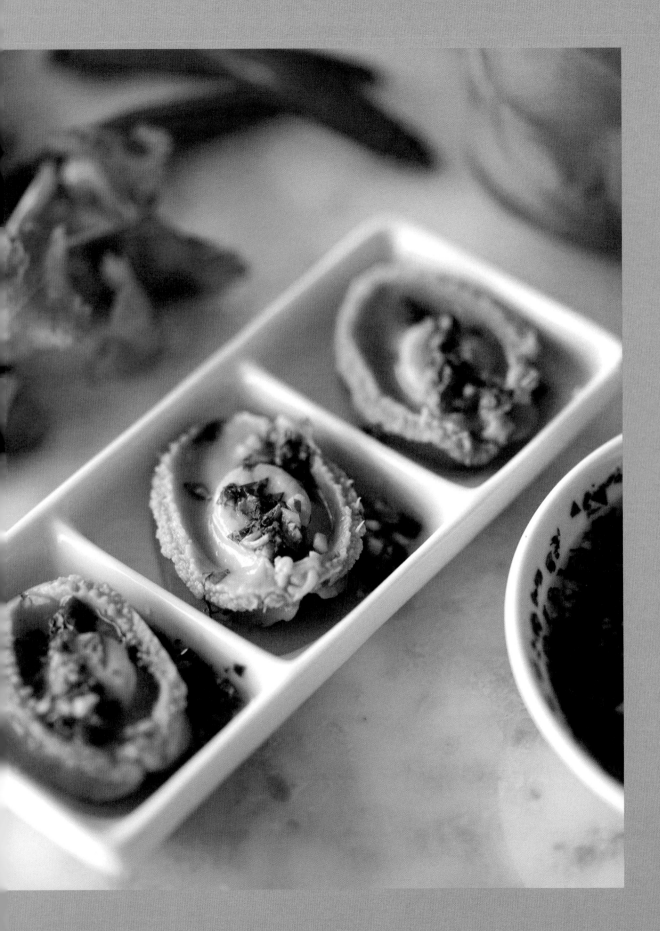

Abalone with Lemon Lime Spicy Sauce

Abalone is a shellfish that is considered an exotic ingredient. Its meat is flavorful and is very high in protein. If abalone is not available, you can substitute other shellfish instead. The Lemon Lime Spicy Sauce will go well with other ingredients such as cooked prawns, squids, clams...

Ingredients

Canned Abalone	(about 8-12 pcs a can)
Rock Sugar	1 tsp
Black Sesame	1 pinch

Sauce

Lemon Lime Spicy Sauce (p.036)	1 portion

Method

1. Drain abalone from the can, discard the juice.

2. Transfer abalone to an airtight glass jar; and put a tsp of rock sugar in the jar.

3. Fill the jar with distilled water. Make sure the abalone is covered by the liquid. This will take away the saltiness from the brine. This step can be prepared days ahead.

4. Take abalone out from the jar and score on the side where the 'pillow' is.

5. To plate, place abalone on a plate and spoon sauce over them.

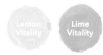

Chinese Recipe p.123

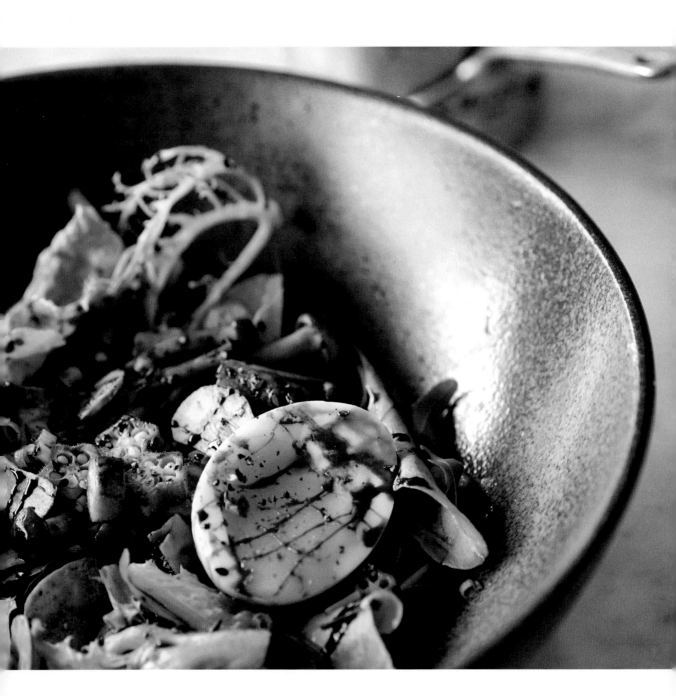

Asian Fungi Salad

Mushrooms & Fungi are flavorful and they add to a simple salad more texture. They are often low in calories, low in sodium & fat free. They are also packed with fiber, vitamins and minerals.

Ingredients

Soft boiled egg	1
Wood Ear Fungus	1oz
Shimeji Mushroom	1oz
Shitake Mushroom, cut in quarters	1oz
Okra, diced	2-3
Ghee	1 tsp
Tamari or Soy Sauce	1 tsp
Salad Greens	handful
Black Sesame Seeds	½ tsp
Garlic, thinly sliced	1 clove
Extra Virgin Olive Oil	2 tbsp
Grapefruit Balsamic Glaze (p.035)	drizzle

Method

1. Make boiling water in a pot enough to cover an egg. When water boils, slowly lower an egg of room temperature and let it boil for 6 minutes. Take it out and run in under cold water. When it is completely cooled, carefully peel off the shell.

2. Wash and drain greens. Poach the okra and set aside.

3. In a pan, warm the olive oil in low heat. Fry garlic slices until just slightly browned. Place them on a paper towel. They will darken afterwards. Pour the olive oil into your serving bowl and swirl it around in order to coat the inside of the bowl. Place greens into the bowl and mix.

4. In a heated pan, add ghee and stir fry all the fungus and mushrooms for 2-3 minutes. Season with tamari and black pepper. Place funghi on top of the greens.

5. To serve, cut the egg in half and place on top of the greens. Drizzle Grapefruit Balsamic Glaze over and sprinkle with sesame seeds and garlic slices to finish.

Grapefruit Vitality

Chinese Recipe p.123

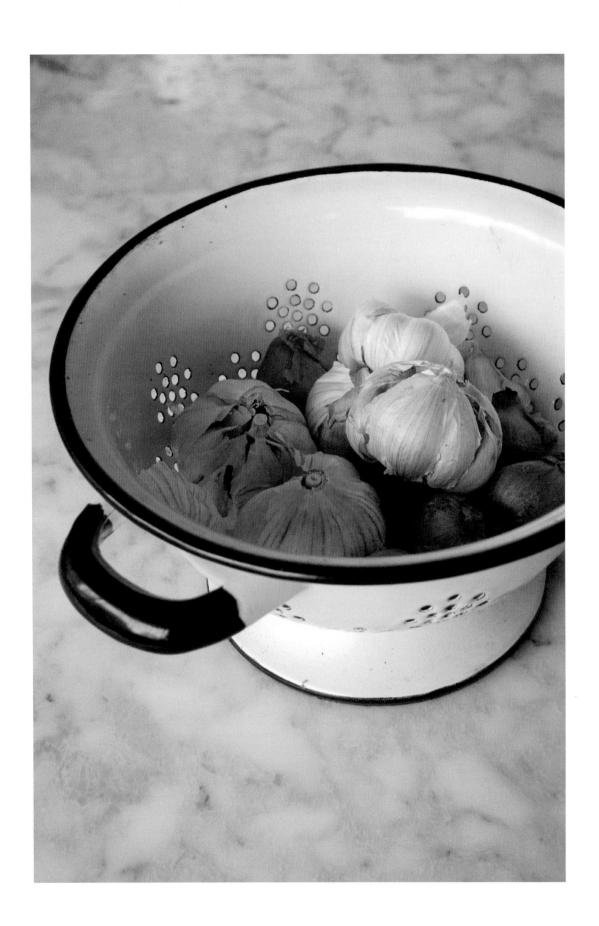

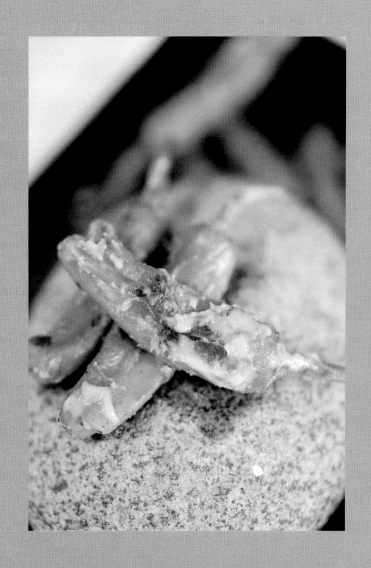

To eat is a necessity,
but to eat intelligently is an art.

Roasted Shishito Peppers with Jade Lemon Fermented Beancurd Paste

Don't be scared with the word Shishito, I can never pronounce it right either. How often do things happen in the exact right way, anyway? I'm just going go with the flow and trust my intuition. Today my intuition tells me I want something cheesy, but knowing I prefer to stay away from dairy... I opt for the chinese fermented beancurd which also gives that irresistible gooey and cheesy feel.

Ingredients

Shishito Peppers	12 pieces approx
Jade Lemon Fermented Beancurd Sauce (p.036)	1 tbsp
Tahini	1 tbsp

Method

1. In a hot pan/ cast iron griddle over the stove top, char shishito peppers. This is ready when the skin of the peppers start to burn.

2. Mix together the Jade Lemon Fermented Beancurd Sauce with the tahini.

3. Slather the mixture on peppers.

4. Garnish with bonito flakes.

Jade Lemon Vitality

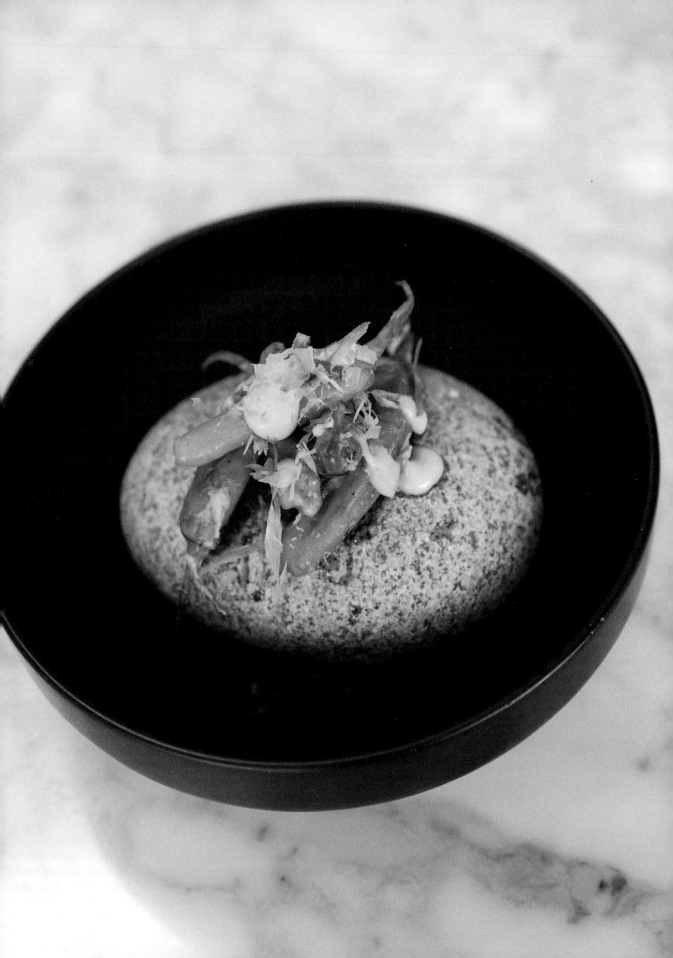

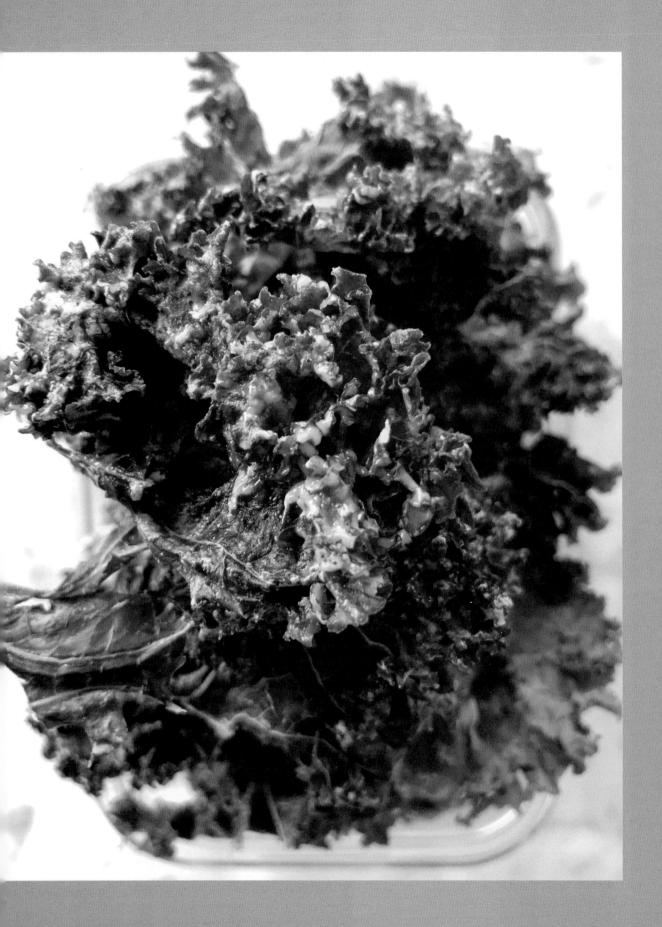

Kale Chips

Of all the superfoods, Kale is my favourite. That's why even if everyone has their own Kale Chips recipe, I decided I have to have my own too! What has made this recipe special is the intense flavous coming from the vitality oils and the very Asian White Miso. Try it & you'll believe it.

Ingredients

Kale	1 big bunch

Dressing Recipe 1

Soaked cashews	½ cup
Pine nuts	¼ cup
Lemon Vitality™	8 drops
Garlic, minced	1 clove
White Miso	2 tbsp
Black Pepper	½ tsp
Dulse Flakes, finely chopped	1 tsp (optional)
Olive oil	2 tbsp
Water, for thinning the consistency	¼ cup
Salt	pinch
Chilli Paste	1 tsp (optional)

Dressing Recipe 2

Olive Oil	4 tbsp
Garlic, minced	1 clove
Lemon Vitality™	3 drops
Clove Vitality™	1 drop
Salt	pinch
Pepper	pinch

Method

1. Blend ingredients, saving olive oil until last. Set aside.

2. Tear the leaves off from the kale, massage kale to soften.

3. Add enough dressing to the kale to coat.

4. Dehydrate at 140F for 1.5 hours.

Chinese Recipe p.124

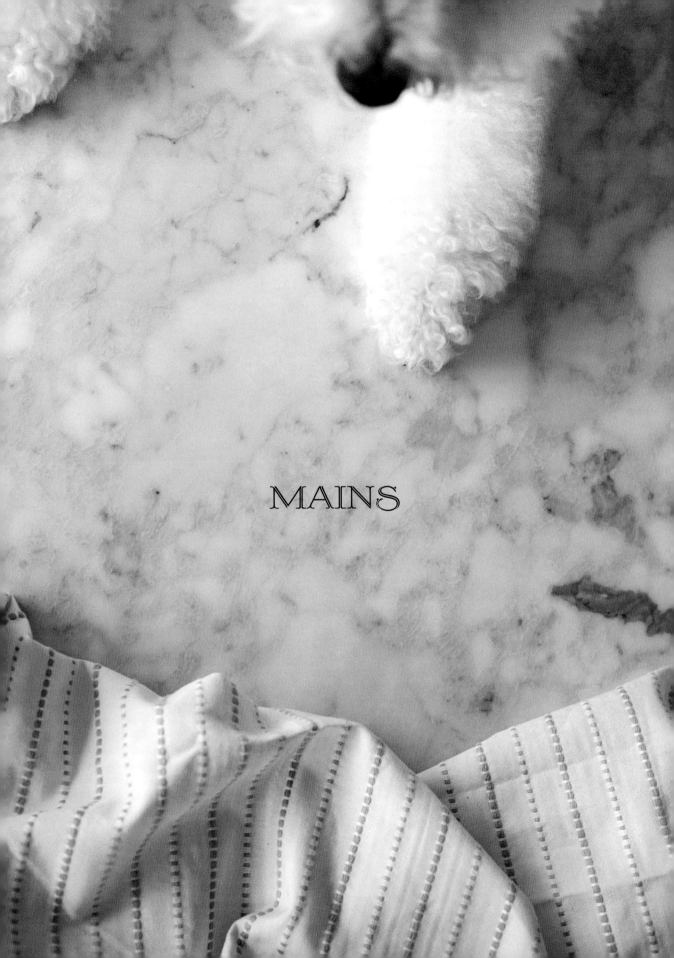

MAINS

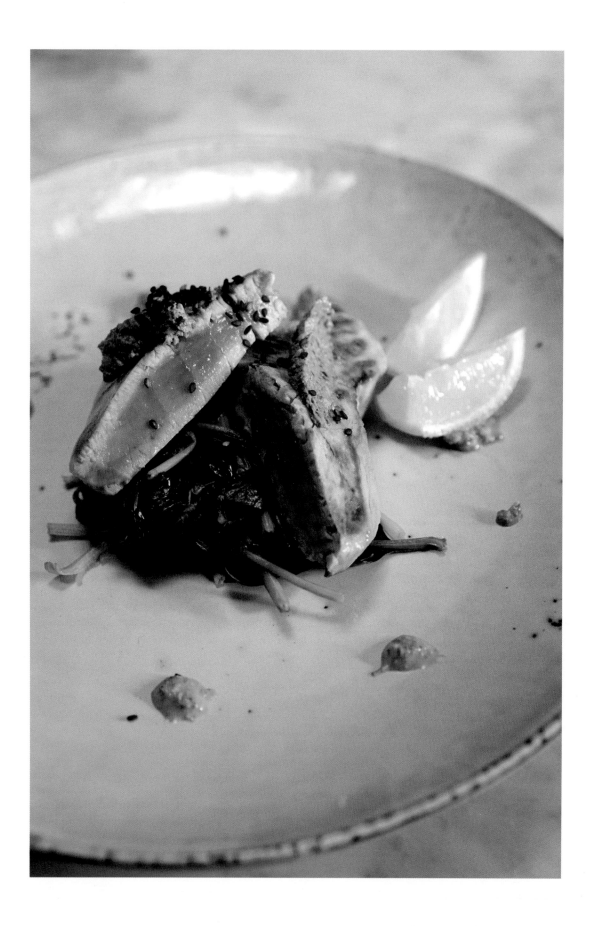

Ahi Tuna Steak Sandwich with Basil Spinach Pesto

I love the versatility of this Spinach Basil Pesto, whether used straight and lathered on fish or stirred into yogurt or coconut cream and served in a wrap, it always hits the spot.

Ingredients

Ahi Tuna Steak	2
Spinach Leaves	2 cups
Basil Spinach Pesto (p.034)	3 tbsp
Olive oil	1 tbsp

Marinade for Ahi Tuna

Olive oil	1 tbsp
Lemon Vitality™	hint
Garlic, crushed	1 clove
Tamari	1 tbsp
Agave	½ tbsp

Method

1. Heat 1 tablespoon of olive oil in a pan and sauté spinach leaves until wilted. Add salt and pepper to taste. Set aside.

2. Sear both sides of the ahi tuna steaks in a pan with medium high heat. It should take 1 minute on each side. (Depending on the desired doneness, adjust the time.)

3. To serve, plate wilted spinach in the center of a plate. Place ahi tuna on top and put a dollop of Basil Spinach Pesto on top. Garnish with black sesame seeds.

4. You can also mix Basil Spinach Pesto with some olive oil to make a looser sauce for drizzling.

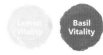

Chinese Recipe p.124

Black Pepper Tomato Beef Goulash

If you have made black pepper sauce from scratch, you'll know how much black pepper you'll need in order to extract that distinct flavor of these tiny peppers. With Black Pepper Vitality, making the sauce becomes a breeze.

In this recipe, I've added a tomato based sauce to make a goulash. But if you want to use the black pepper sauce alone, it pairs beautifully with meats such as chicken or beef too.

Ingredients

Beef Fillet, thickly sliced	2 lbs
(I use USDA grass fed beef)	
Arrowroot Flour	3 tbsp
Tomato, diced	2
Green Pepper, thinly sliced	1
Button Mushrooms, sliced	10-12
Tomato Paste	2 tbsp
Paprika	¼ tsp
Beef Stock	¾ cup
Wine	¼ cup
Mustard	2 tsp
Coconut Cream/ Sour Cream	5 oz
Tamari	½ tsp
Salt	Pinch
Parsley	Bunch
Cooking Oil	2 tbsp
Nutmeg Vitality™	2 drops
Black Pepper Sauce (p.034)	1 portion of the recipe

Method

1. Heat a casserole dish and add a tablespoon of oil.

2. Sprinkle the beef with flour and add to the casserole to brown. When the beef is browned, take it out and set aside.

3. In the same casserole dish, add another tablespoon of oil; then add in the green pepper to stir fry until softened; followed by the button mushrooms. Deglaze with some wine. Continue to cook the vegetables until softened, and set aside.

4. Return the beef to the casserole and add in the beef stock, tomato puree, paprika, mustard, tamari and Nutmeg Vitality. Cook for 25 minutes.

5. Return the green pepper and button mushrooms to the casserole and cook for another 5 minutes.

6. To serve, stir in coconut cream or sour cream; and sprinkle parsley on top.

Chinese Recipe p.124 ➤

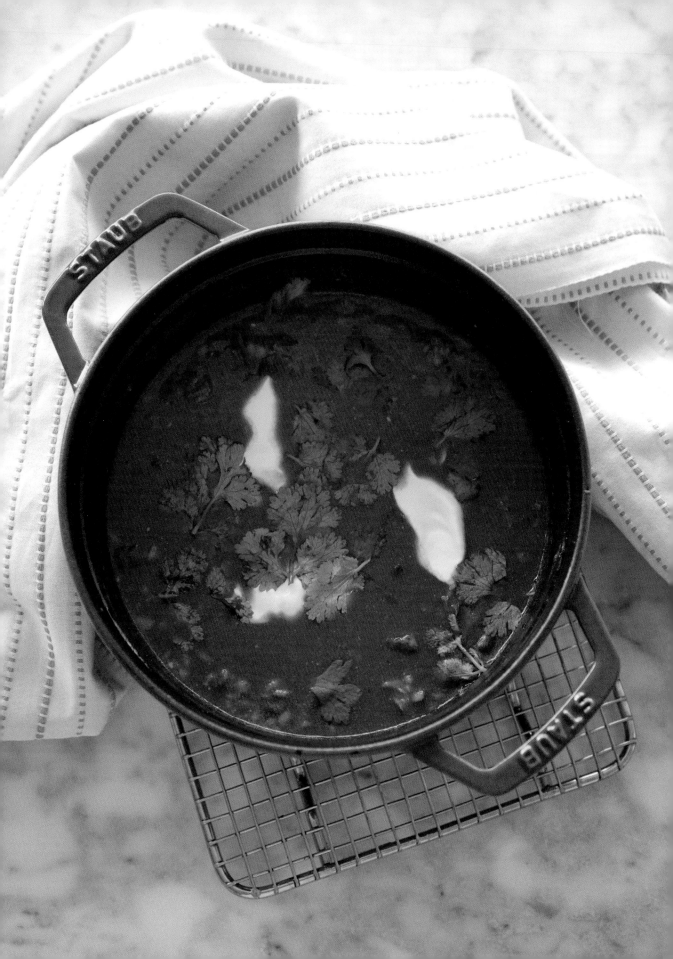

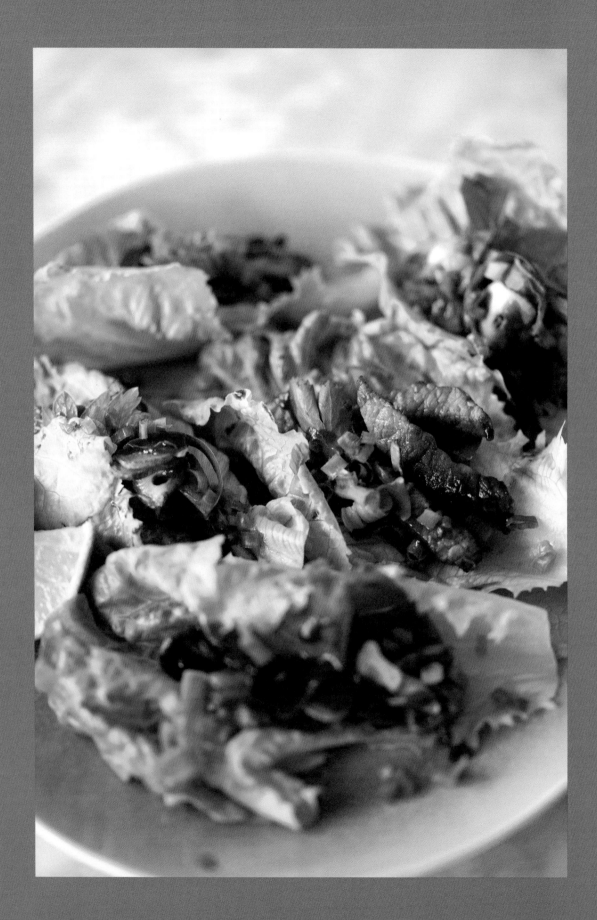

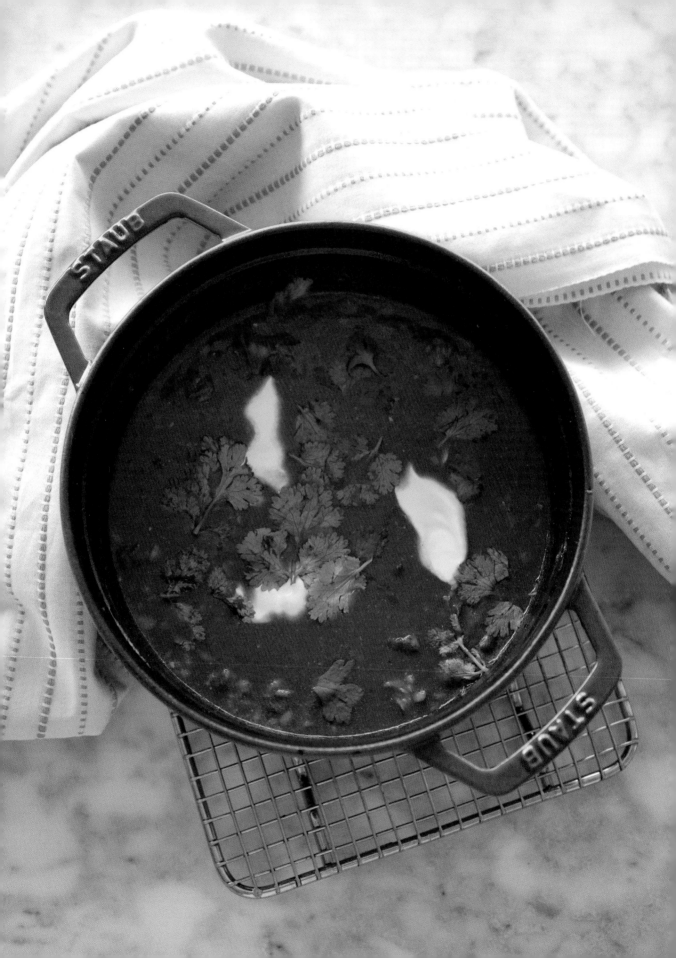

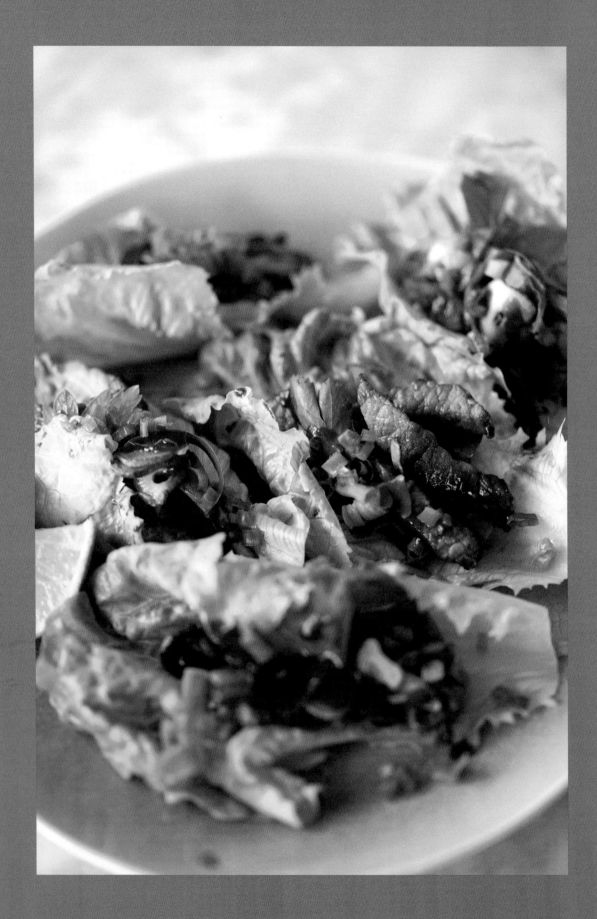

Citrus Fresh Gojujang Pork Lettuce Wrap

Pork lettuce wraps are a fun and adventurous way to introduce new flavors to your guests. These sumptuous wraps are a lot like tacos; they're finger foods you can easily pick up and are very fast to make. Don't let this little amount of sauce disguise you. It is spicy, tangy & finger licking good.

Ingredients

Pork Collar, julienne	5oz
Garlic, cut into think slices	1 clove
Lettuce	4-5 leaves
Shiso Leaf / Parsley	handful
Spring Onion	2 stalks
Citrus Fresh Gojujang Sauce (p.035)	4 tbsp
Cooking Oil	2 tbsp

Method

1. Cut spring onion into two sections: the white end being 2" long, the rest chopped.

2. In a hot iron pan, heat some cooking oil.

3. When it's slightly warm, place the sliced garlic in the pan and heat until it's golden. Remove the garlic slices from the pan and place on a kitchen towel to soak off excess oil.

4. In the same pan, fry the white part if the spring onion until fragrant.

5. Put the pork collar in the pan to cook. The pan should now be very hot and the pork will char. When the pork is 70% cooked, add in half of the Citrus Fresh Gojujang Sauce and continue to let the pork cook.

6. To serve, arrange lettuce on a plate, put shiso leaf on top of the lettuce followed by the pork. Drizzle with more sauce and sprinkle with chopped spring onion/parsley on top.

Citrus Fresh Vitality

Chinese Recipe p.125

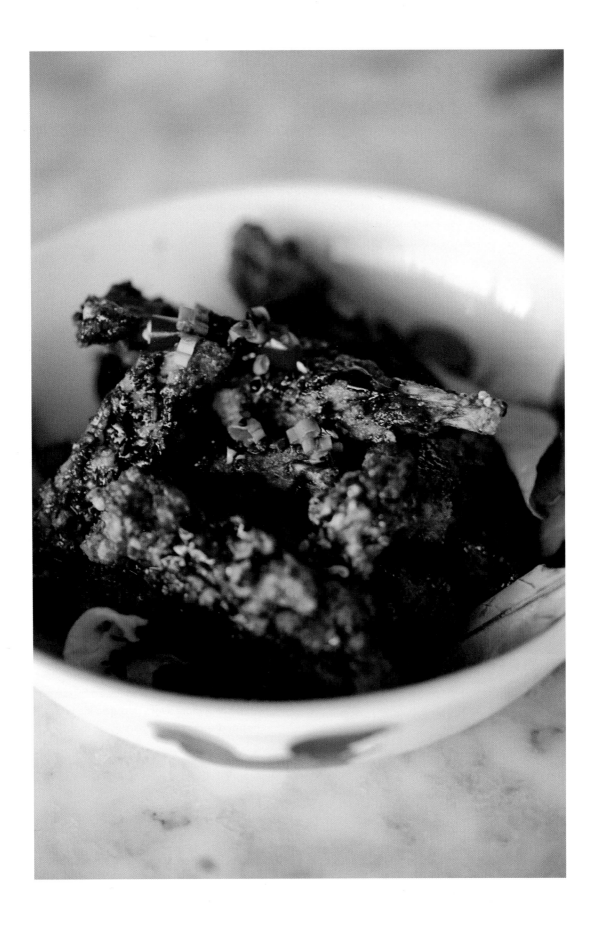

Fried Chicken Wings with Spicy Balsamic Glaze

I have a thing for fried chicken wings. They are so finger licking good, sometimes I can eat a whole plate just by myself! This time, when I'm about to smack my face into yet another plate of goodness, I decided to whip up a version that makes it guilt-free.

Thanks to the availability of these hormone-free chicken wings from my neighborhood grocery store, I decided to take my grapefruit balsamic glaze and kick it up with tamari and honey. For those who like some spicyness, add in chilli flakes or red chili oil too!!

Ingredients

Mid Joint Chicken Wings	10 pieces
Ginger Vitality™	3 drops
Shaoxing Wine	1 tbsp
Egg	1
Eikorn Flour	5 tbsp
Garlic Powder	1 tsp
Onion Powder	1 tsp
Essential Oil Infused Balsamic Glaze	1 portion
(p.035) *(I choose Grapefruit Vitality for this recipe)*	
Raw Honey	1 tbsp
Tamari or Soy Sauce	¼ tsp
Red Chili Oil	¼ tsp
Crushed Peanuts or Sesame for garnish	optional
Cooking Oil	¾ cup

Tips

* Cranking up the heat at the end of a deep frying process will take out the greasiness from the deep fry.

Chinese Recipe p.125

Method

1. Clean and pat dry chicken wings. Cut vertically so each piece has just one bone.

2. Marinade with Ginger Vitality and shaoxing wine for 15 minutes.

3. Drain chicken wings from excess marinade.

4. Set up a flour dredging station: whisk one egg and place in a bowl; in another bowl or plate, stir together flour, garlic powder and onion powder. Dip chicken wings in egg first, then dredge chicken with flour mixture and pat off excess.

5. Deep fry them in hot oil in medium heat. This will take about 2 minutes, make sure you flip them once in between. Take the chicken wings out. Adjust the heat to high and finish frying for another 30 - 45 seconds. Take them out and place on kitchen paper to absorb excess oil.

6. Meanwhile, put the grapefruit balsamic glaze in a bowl and stir it together with honey, tamari, red chili oil.

7. Place chicken wings in the bowl and toss them with the balsamic glaze.

8. To serve, sprinkle with red chili flakes, sesame seeds or spring onion.

General Tsao Spicy Sticky Chicken

Get ready for an unbelieveable juicy & impressive chicken dish!

This lighter version of General Tsao chicken is made with a combination of Tangerine, Thyme, and Ginger essential oils. Try serving this on a sizzling hot plate, it will help the sauce to caramelize making it sticky and finger licking good.

Ingredients

Chicken Thigh	3 pieces
Arrowroot Flour / Tapioca Flour	2 tbsp
Cooking Oil	1 tbsp
Shallots, sliced	3 pcs
Spring Onion	2 stalks
Sesame seeds	Sprinkle

Marinade

Shaoxing Wine	1 tbsp
Soy Sauce/ Tamari	1 tsp
White Pepper	½ tsp

Sauce

Tangerine Thyme Sticky Sauce (p.039)	1 portion
Chicken Stock or Water	3 tbsp

Method

1. Mix together the ingredients for the marinade and marinade the chicken thighs for 15-20 minutes.

2. Take chicken out from the marinade and slightly pat dry.

3. Dredge flour over the chicken pieces.

4. In a heated pan, add in the cooking oil.

5. Sweat spring onion and shallots until fragrant, push aside.

6. Add chicken thigh, skin side down, to the pan and pan fry for about 6 minutes. Turn over the chicken when the skin has browned. Continue to cook the meat side for another 3 minutes or until it comes off from the pan easily.

7. Meanwhile, mix the remaining marinade with 3 tbsp water/stock.

8. Add the sauce to the pan. Cover with lid and turn heat down to a simmer. There should be enough liquid to braise the chicken, but not too much that the skin is covered in liquid.

9. Simmer for 15 minutes in medium heat or until chicken is cooked through.

10. The sauce should be thick and glossy. If the sauce is not thick enough, take the chicken out and set aside. Then turn up and heat and reduce the sauce until thickened.

11. To serve spoon some sauce over chicken and sprinkle with sesame seeds and spring onion.

Tangerine Vitality   Thyme Vitality   Ginger Vitality

Chinese Recipe p.126 ➜

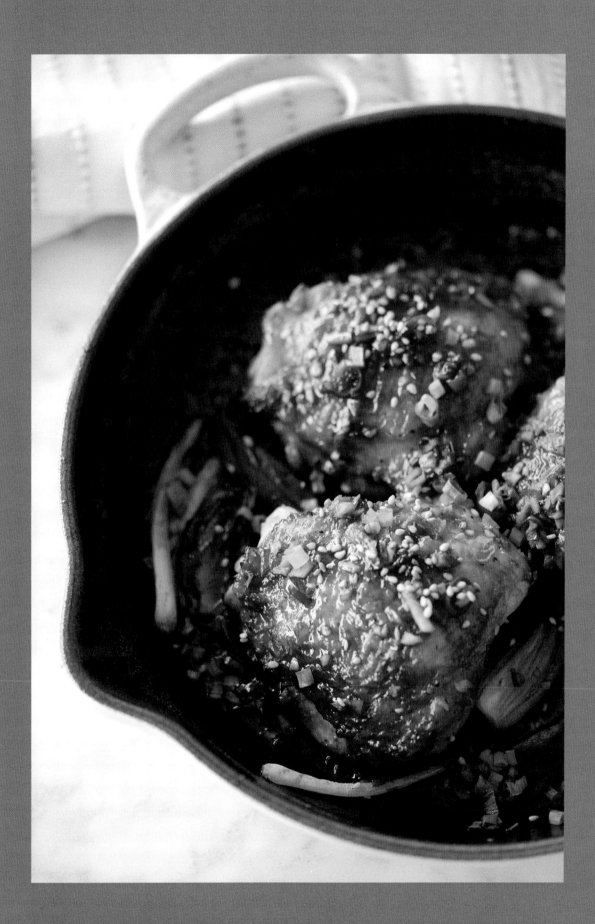

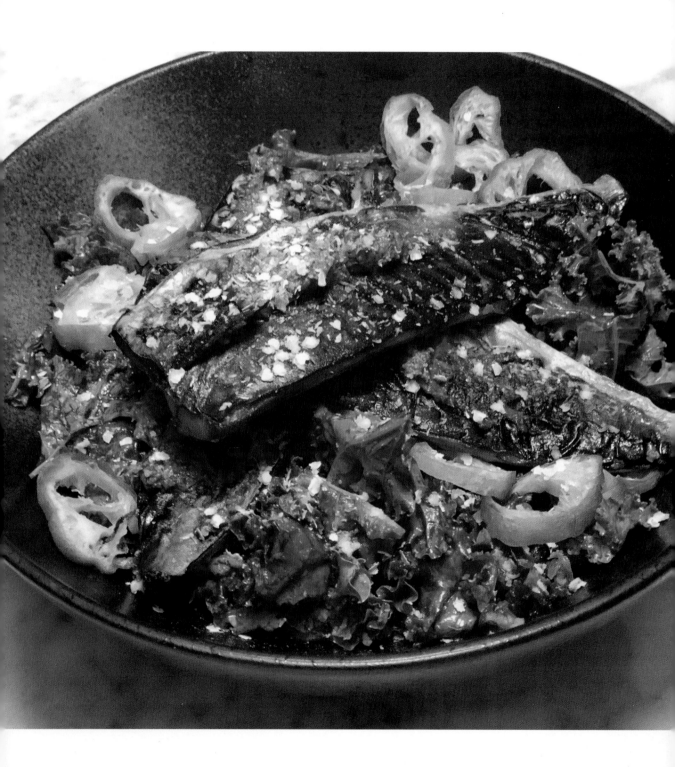

Grilled Mackerel with Wasabi Citrus Fresh Salsa Verde

This is a dish where everything is very simply seasoned. The kick to it is the Salsa Verde, which is packed with flavors that will certainly awaken your palette. Just like life, sometimes you let things be and enjoy the solitude; other times live your life with a little spice.

Ingredients

Mackerel Fillet	2
Salt	1 tsp
Olive oil	½ tbsp
Wasabi Citrus Fresh Salsa Verde (p.039)	½ portion

Method

1. Clean and wash the mackerel fillet. Pat dry with a kitchen towel.

2. Sprinkle the salt on the meat side of the fish.

3. Brush the olive oil on the skin side of the fish, sprinkle with more salt on the skin side.

4. Line a roasting pan with aluminum foil. Place fish fillet on the pan with skin side up.

5. Roast in a preheated oven on the upper rack at 180C for 10-15 minutes or until the skin is crispy & browned.

6. To serve, put a spoonful of salsa verde on top of the grilled mackerel. Drizzle with more olive oil if desired. Top with croutons or chinese fried dough.

Tips

* Mix a simple Kale Salad and dress with olive oil, lemon juice, salt, and minced garlic. Top with pomegranate and quinoa flakes.

* Break off the hard stalks from the kale, leaving just the leaves. Massage the leaves until they're softened. This salad can be prepared 2-3 hours ahead of time.

Citrus Fresh Vitality   Lemon Vitality

Chinese Recipe p.126 ➤

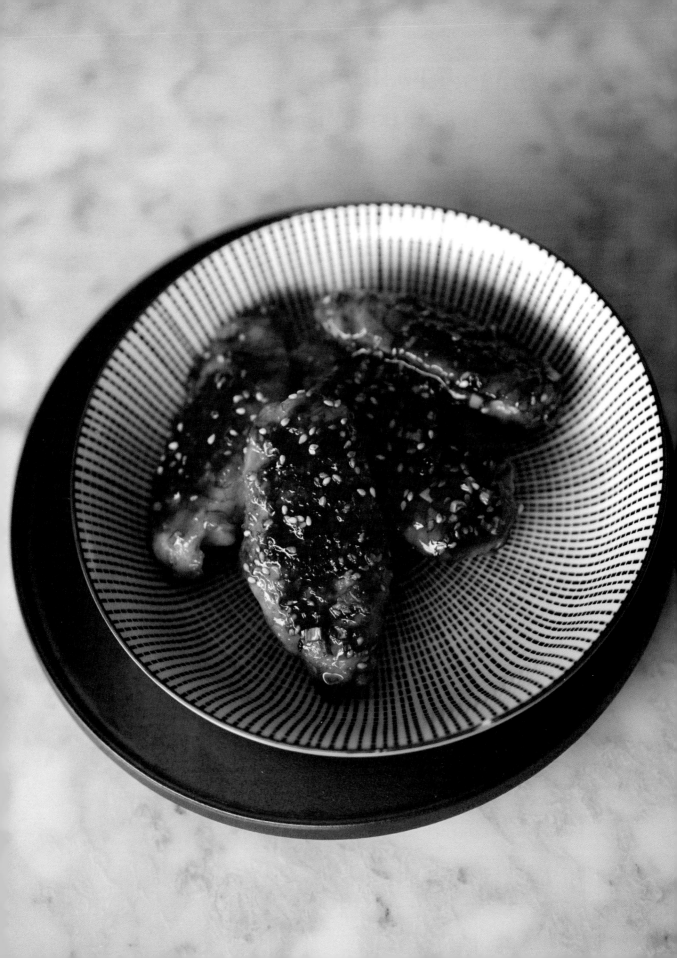

Soy Jade Lemon Chicken Wings

There are so many ways to season chicken wings; and the good thing is - they always turn out delicious. I have used Jade Lemon Vitality oil here to take off some heaviness of the wings; but really you can play around with different flavors to suit your taste. After all, cooking goes by sense, taste and instinct. And the kitchen is the best place to demonstrate that! My kitchen is for dancing, how about yours?

Ingredients

Chicken Wings Mid Joint	8
Soy Jade Lemon Butter Sauce (p.038)	1 portion
Toasted White Sesame	2 tbsp
Spring Onion, chopped	1 tbsp
Arrowroot Flour / Tapioca Flour	4 tbsp
Cooking Oil	1 tbsp
Honey	2 tbsp

Method

1. Wash and pat dry chicken wings.

2. Dredge chicken wings with flour and pan fry them in 1 tablespoon of hot oil until both sides are golden brown. Check to see if they're cooked through by inserting a chopstick in the middle. If there is no sight of blood from the chicken wings, that means they're cooked.

3. While chicken wings are cooking in the pan; stir the honey and sesame seeds into the sauce and mix well.

4. When the chicken wings are fully cooked, turn the heat off and pour in the honey sauce mixture, immediately followed by the spring onion. Toss quickly so the wings are generously coated with the sauce.

Jade Lemon Vitality

Chinese Recipe p.126 ▶

Jade Lemon Fermented Beancurd Lamb Belly Stew

The time to eat lamb at its absolute best is in the autumn and winter of the year. At home, stewed lamb is often seasoned with fermented beancurd and kaffir lime leaves. It is always a dish shared amongst the family which brings back a lot of sweet memories.

I hope this lamb stew will do the same for you.

Ingredients

Lamb Belly	18 oz
Chinese Sweet Bean Paste	3 tbsp
Jade Lemon Fermented Beancurd Sauce (p.036)	1 portion
Water Chestnut, peeled and cut in halves	6
White Turnip, cut into chunks	½
Beancurd Sheets	1-2 sheets
Cooking Oil	1 tbsp
Shaoxing Wine	1 tbsp
Ginger	2 slices
Dark Soy Sauce	2 tsp
Sugar	½ tbsp
Arrowroot Flour	1 tsp + 1 tbsp water
Water	1-2 cups

Method

1. Bring a pot of water to a boil. Blanch the lamb belly for 10 minutes. Take lamb belly out and discard the water. Set aside lamb belly.

2. Add 1 tbsp of oil to a casserole, when oil is heated, add in the ginger.

3. Add in the lamb belly, and brown the sides. Splash in the shaoxing wine.

4. Add in the Chinese sweet bean paste and Jade Lemon Beancurd Sauce ,mix well.

5. Add in water chestnut and enough water to cover. Let it simmer for 30 minutes.

6. Add in the turnips, beancurd sheets and simmer for another 10 minutes.

7. Add dark soy sauce and sugar to taste.

8. In a small bowl, mix together arrowroot flour and 1 tbsp of water to make a slurry.

9. Add the slurry to the lamb, and turn up the heat to a boil. Meanwhile keep stirring until the simmering soup comes to a sauce consistency.

10. To serve, top with cilantro.

Jade Lemon Vitality

Chinese Recipe p.127

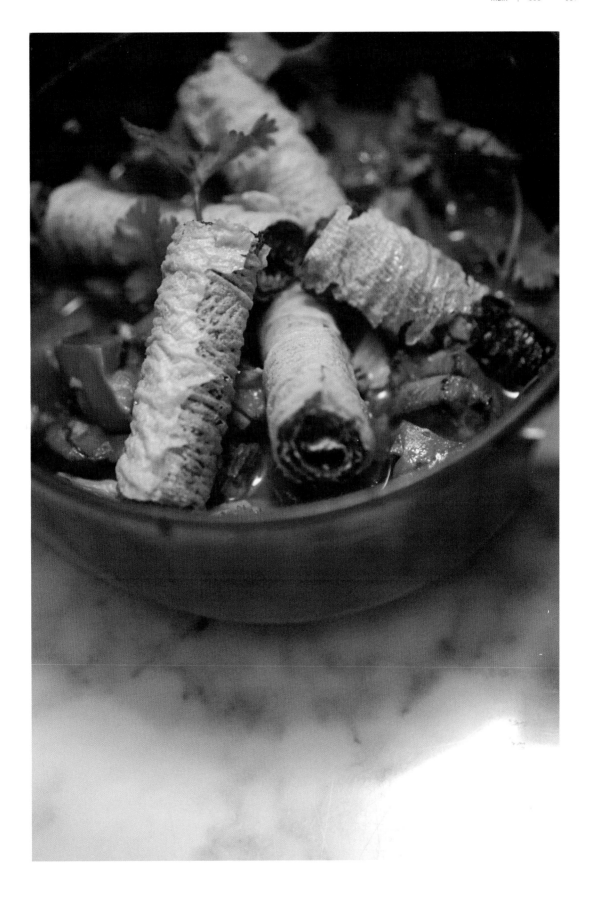

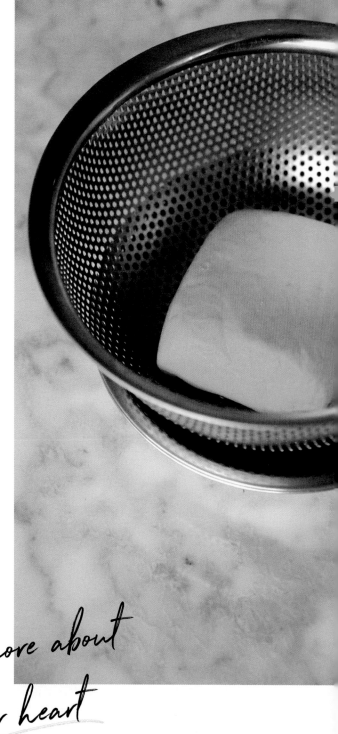

Real cooking is more about
following your heart
than following recipes.

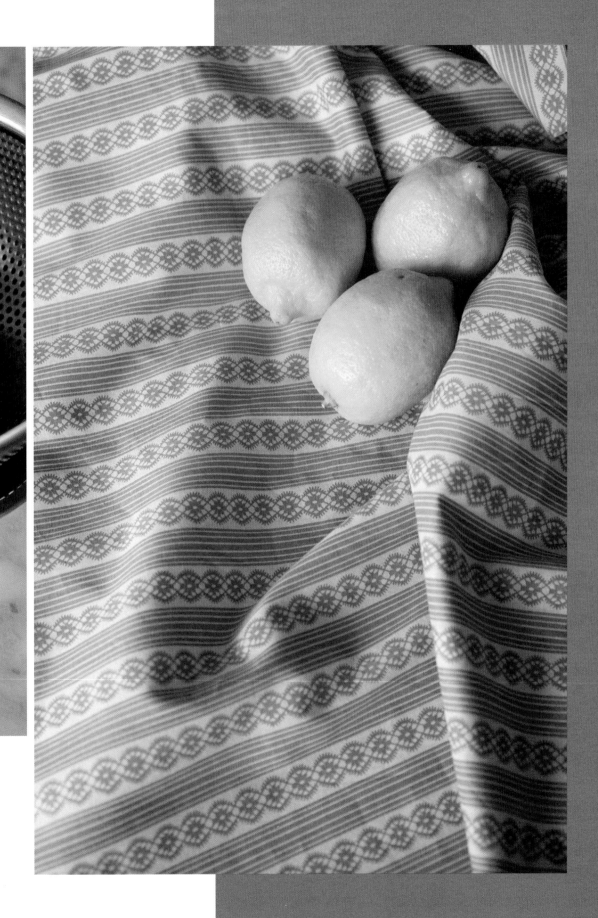

Lemon Lime Mexican Noodle Soup

This lemon lime noodle soup is a remake based on a dish called the lima chicken soup, originated from Mexico. The first time I tried it, I was fascinated by the complex flavors of it. When I tried to taste the flavors separately, it was sweet, spicy, salty and tangy. Yet when these flavors are combined, they strike a perfect balance, making it interesting and super delicious. Which reminds me of a Chinese saying, that life is made up of sweetness, tanginess, bitterness & spiciness. When you are going through the taste of it separately, you might be wondering what's going on. Yet when at a point when you look back in life, you realize it is because of these moments that have made life so interesting and perfect.

Ingredients

| Tofu Cream |

Firm Tofu	4oz
Olive oil	1 tsp
Salt	pinch of salt to taste

| Noodle Soup |

Yellow Onion, sliced	½
Garlic, minced	2 cloves
Olive oil	1 tbsp
Chicken Breast	2 pcs
Chicken Broth	3 cups
Roma Tomatoes, diced	4
Oregano Vitality™	1 drop
Lemon Lime Spicy Sauce (p.036)	3-4 tbsp
Parsley, chopped	small bunch
Chili, diced	1-2 (optional)
Salt	pinch
Rice noodle	portion for 2
Fresh Lime	1

Tips

* The original recipe calls for avocado, which magically adds creaminess to the soup and balance off the sharp flavors from the ingredients. For those who opt for something other than avocado, I suggest adding a good dollop of this tofu cream.

Method

| Tofu Cream | *(Can be prepared a day ahead of time)*

1. Place all ingredients in a blender, process until very creamy and smooth (about 1 minute).

2. Refrigerate for at least an hour to thicken.

| Noodle Soup |

1. In a pot with medium heat, sweat onion and garlic with olive oil.

2. Add diced tomatoes and chicken broth and bring to a simmer.

3. In a separate pot, steam chicken until cooked through. About 10-15 minutes.

4. When chicken is cooked through and cool enough to handle, pull the meat apart.

5. Add the Lemon Lime Spicy Sauce to the boiling soup. Put rice noodles to the soup to cook, about 8 minutes.

6. When the noodle is cooked, divide into two bowls. Put chicken on top of noodles and ladle soup into the bowl.

7. Add half an avocado or a dollop of tofu sour cream and sprinkle parsley on top, and finish a squeeze of lime.

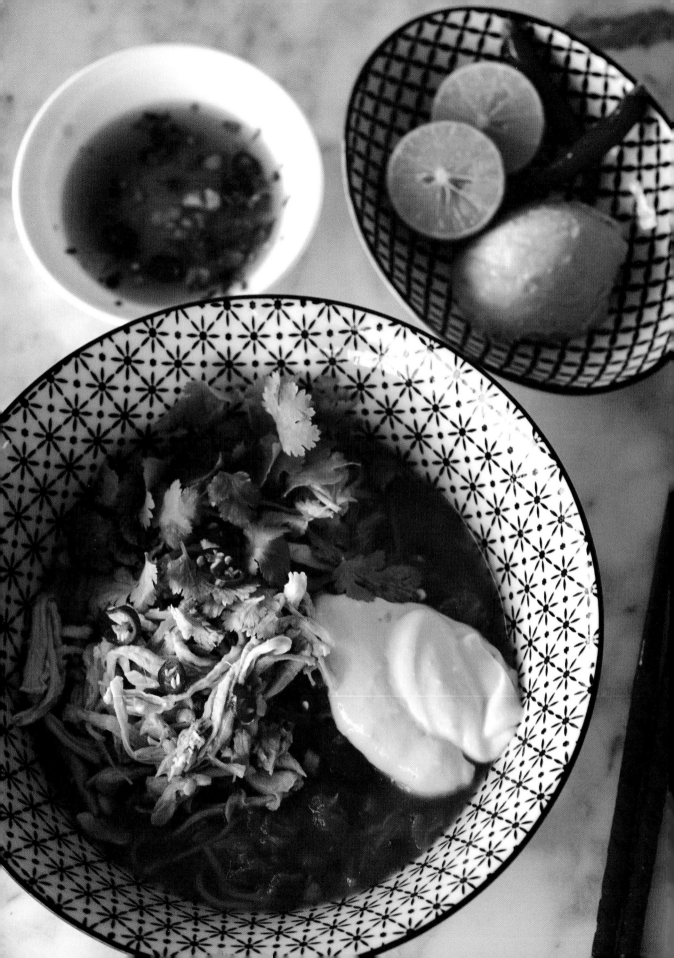

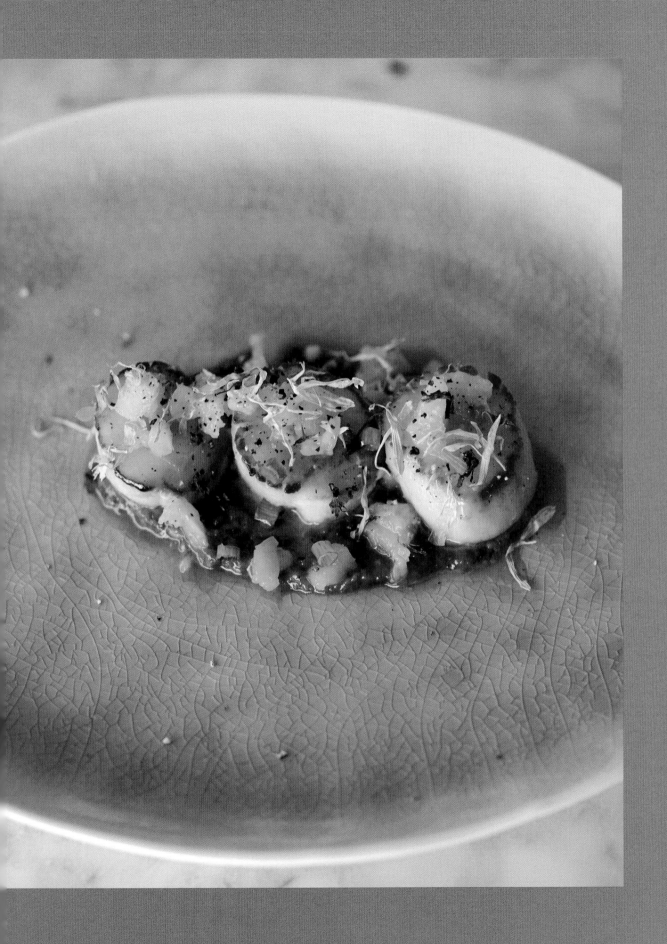

Lemongrass Scented Fermented Rice Sauce with Scallop

The coconut cream provides a perfect platform on which a fresh fruity and tropical sauce is built. Reminiscing a pina colada cocktail, you will be pleasantly surprised to find a hint of lemongrass flavor throughout.

Ingredients

Scallops	6
(I use frozen large sized sashimi grade scallops)	
Coconut Cream	4 tbsp
Chicken Stock	2 tbsp
Agave	½ tbsp
Ghee/Butter	1 knob
Cooking Oil	2 tbsp
Pineapple, diced	4 wedges
Fermented Rice Sauce	1 portion
Lemongrass Vitality™	hint

Method

1. Add to the Fermented Rice Sauce the coconut cream, agave and chicken stock, and mix well.

2. In a pan, heat up a little oil and sauté the pineapple dices for just 10 seconds, then set aside.

3. For the scallops, melt the butter with some cooking oil in high heat. When the butter is melted, pan fry the scallops on both sides. You want the sides caramelized but not over cooked. This will take about 1 ½ minutes on each side. Take out & set aside.

4. Deglaze the same pan with the fermented rice sauce mixture. The sauce will turn brown picking up all the yumminess from the pan.

5. To serve, spoon sauce on the bottom of a plate. Put scallops on top and decorate with pineapple dices.

6. Drizzle with olive oil or decorate with edible flowers.

Chinese Recipe p.127

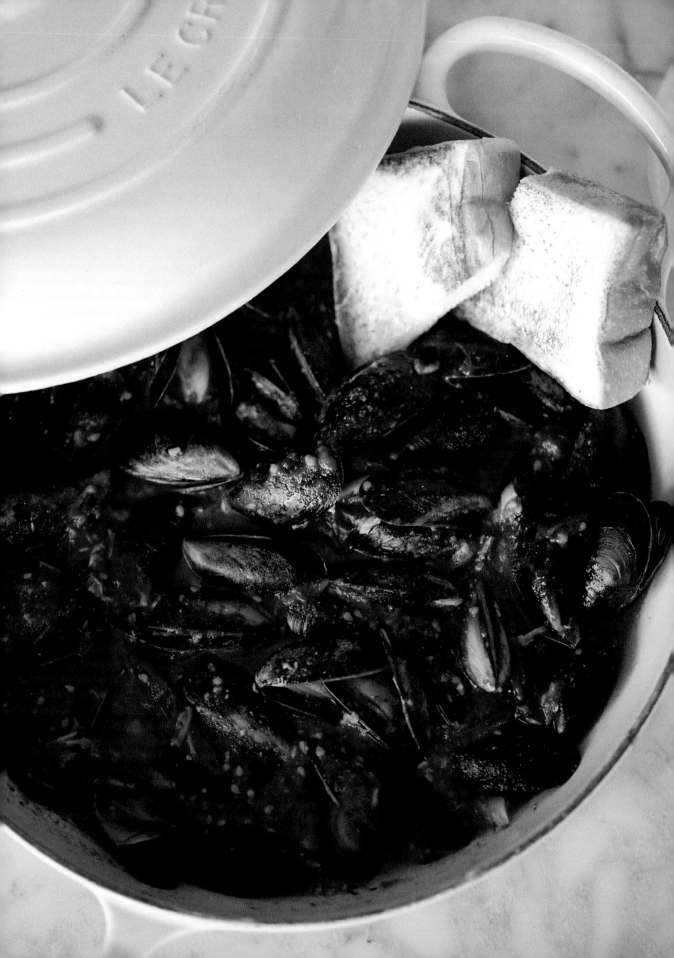

Mussels in Tomato Lemongrass

Mussels are sold live and frozen as whole cooked or raw. I am using frozen raw blue mussels which have a distinctive rich, sweet taste and are complemented well in various sauces. In this recipe, I have enhanced a basic tomato sauce with Lemongrass Vitality. The flavor of the lemongrass is quite light and does not overpower the rest of flavors. Afterall, it is all about striking a balance, right?

Ingredients

| Tomato Sauce |

Roma tomato	14 oz
(I use the small ones on vine which are more flavorful)	
Garlic	4 cloves
Onion Powder	1 tsp
Garlic Powder	1 tsp
Dried Thyme	1 tsp
Salt	pinch
White wine/ Vodka/ Sake/ Stock	⅓ cup
Fermented Rice Sauce	1 tbsp
Lemongrass Vitality™	hint
Frozen Blue Mussels	1 lb
Eikorn Pasta	handful (optional)

Method

1. Take the frozen mussels out from the freezer and let them defrost 20 minutes prior to cooking. Or defrost as suggested on package.

2. Place tomatoes, garlic cloves, onion powder, garlic powder, and thyme together in a pot and bring it to a boil. When the ingredients come to a boil, add in the wine/stock.

3. Turn down the heat to the lowest heat and let it simmer for 30 minutes.

4. When it's done simmering, take out the tomato skin. Mash down the garlic cloves with a spatula against the side of the pot. The sauce is ready and can be set aside.

5. By now, the frozen mussels should have been loosened from the ice rinse, and discard the ice/water.

6. In a pan with medium heat put the mussels in, followed by 1 tbsp of the lemongrass fermented rice sauce. Mix well.

7. Add in all the tomato sauce, stir well.

8. If you are serving pasta with this dish, you can add the pasta in by breaking them into halves by its length.

9. Turn down the heat and let it simmer, covered, for 8 minutes. Stirring once in between.

10. Serve hot.

Chinese Recipe p.128

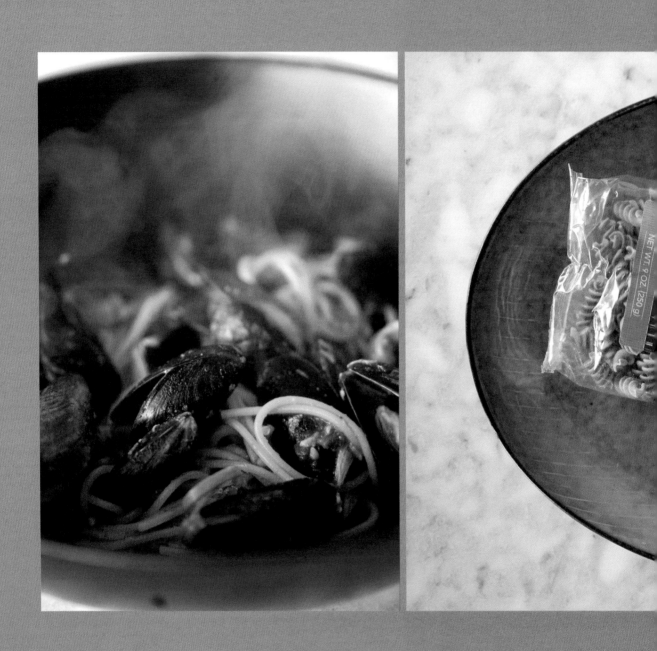

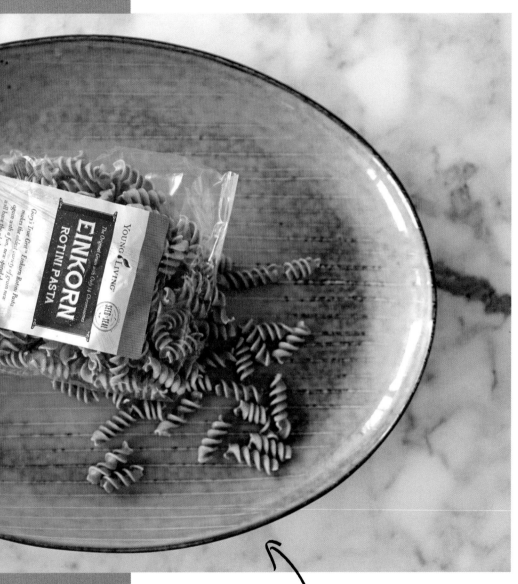

Young Living
Einkorn Rotini Pasta

Pepperish Chicken

This is a lighter take on a dish inspired by a famous local eat from Chiu Chow, which is a city in the GuangDong Province in China. The original dish is rather oily because all ingredients are deep fried including a serving of deep fried greens. The black pepper sauce has been taken to another level when combined with various peppercorns, and the kale chips have magically replaced the deep fried greens.

Pepperish chicken, you just became one of the staple dishes at my home.

Ingredients

Chicken Thigh / Chicken Breast Meat, sliced	1 lb
Cooking Oil	⅓ cup
Ginger	2 slices
Garlic Cloves	2
Red chili, roughly chopped	3-4
Kale Chips (p.051)	(see recipe from snacks)

Marinade *(Optional)*

Soy Sauce / Tamari	2 tsp
Shaoxing Wine	1 tbsp

Sauce

Black Pepper Sauce (p.035)	4 tbsp
Green Peppercorn / Pink Peppercorn	total 4 tsp
Sichuan Peppercorn	

Method

1. In a heated wok with medium heat, add in ⅓ cup of cooking oil.

2. When the oil has reached medium heat, put in the chicken slices and fry until 80% cooked. Move the chicken around so it doesn't stick together. At this point, you are not browning the chicken, instead you're just trying to cook it in gentle heat.

3. Take the chicken out from the wok and set aside.

4. Discard most of the oil, leaving only 2 tbsp.

5. Put in the ginger, garlic and chili; fry until fragrant. Take care not to burn them. Then add in the black pepper sauce, peppercorns; fry until fragrant. This should take just a few seconds.

6. Add the chicken and finish the cooking.

7. To serve, plate chicken on a dish and garnish with kale chips.

Black Pepper Vitality

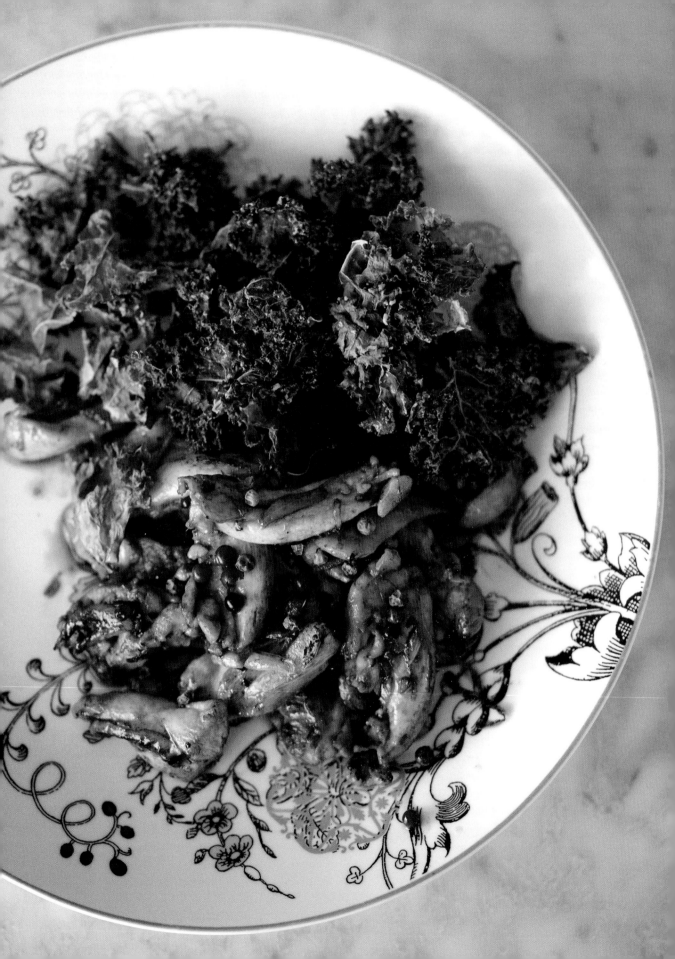

Roast Rack of Lamb with Basil Spinach Pesto

I don't know about you, but cooking and showcasing a dish such as lamb rack always seems so extravagant and festive to me. It is also when you carve the lamb rack and your guests give the 'ohhs and ahhs.'

Nothing brings people together like good food. There's always so much joy and laughter around the dinner table, with everyone smiling... It is simply priceless.

Ingredients

Rack of Lamb	1
Mustard	2 tbsp
(I use French Mustard, you can use Dijon too)	
Basil Spinach Pesto (p.034)	2 tbsp
More Basil Spinach Pesto to serve	1 tbsp
Nut Milk / Olive Oil	1 tbsp

Method

1. Take the lamb rack out from the refrigerator and let it come to room temperature. Cut rack of lamb into two, so each section has 4 rib bones.

2. Stir together the mustard and the basil spinach pesto and slather the mixture all over the rack of lamb. Put the racks fat side up on a baking sheet and let sit for 10 minutes.

3. Preheat oven to 230C. Roast the lamb in the oven for 15 minutes. Turn the oven down to 180C and continue to roast for another 15 minutes.

4. With a meat thermometer, check the internal temperature of the lamb rack. For a medium rare, it should read 60C; for a medium, it should read 68C.

5. When ready, take the lamb racks out from the oven. Put a piece of aluminum foil over the rack and let it sit for 10 minutes before carving.

6. Meanwhile, stir together equal amounts of basil spinach pesto and nut milk or olive oil. Drizzle on top of lamb to serve.

Tips

* Lamb always tastes better with roasted garlic. To roast garlic; cut a head of garlic in half horizontally, drizzle olive oil on top, season with salt and put in the oven together with the lamb rack to roast.

Lemon Vitality
Basil Vitality

Chinese Recipe p.128

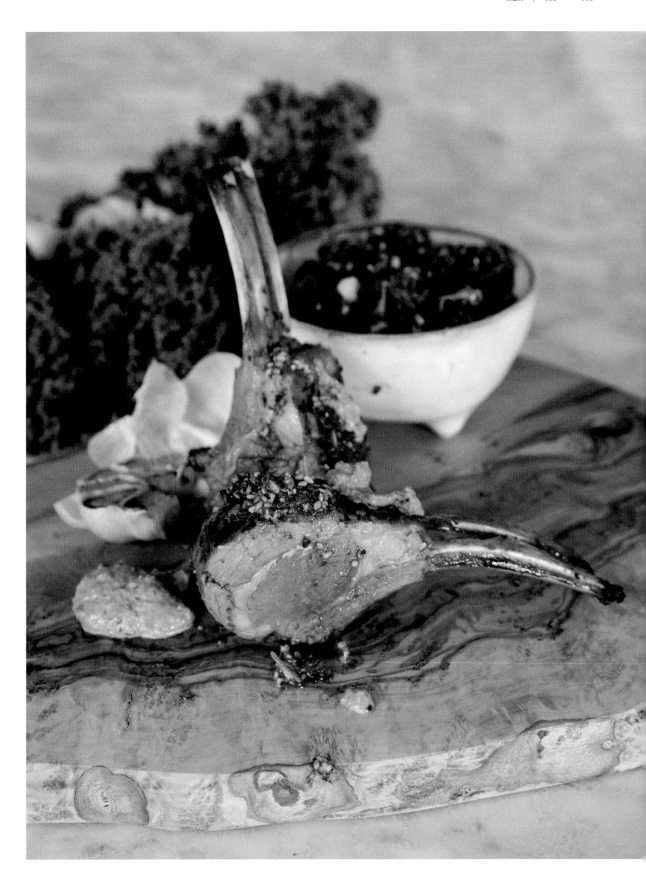

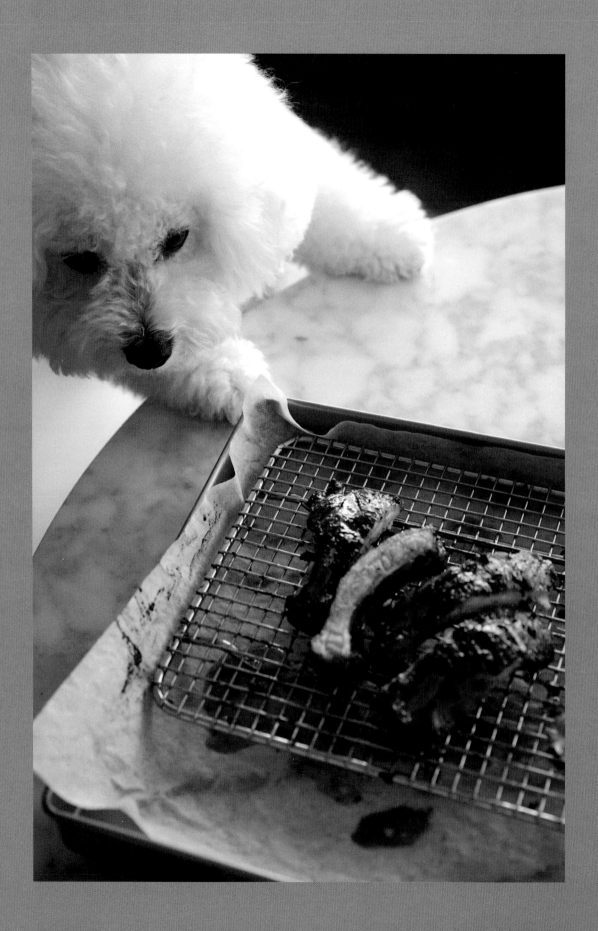

Roasted Orange & Tarragon Spareribs

Sometimes the best things happen when we wait — that is the beauty of fermentation. It requires some planning ahead, but I assure you, this is worth it. The fermentation results in a sauce that has an immense depth and intensity.

The honey Tarragon Vitality and Orange Vitality offsets the richness of the spareribs. Perfect match!

Ingredients

Baby Back Ribs	1 rack of rib

(I buy frozen Danish Pork Ribs)

Marinade

* Prepare this ahead of time as a minimum 8 hour fermentation is required

Sugar	4 tbsp
Salt	½ tbsp
Egg	1
Shallots	2
Garlic	2 cloves
Head of Chinese Celery	1 stalk
Fermented Black Bean, minced	1 tbsp
Chinese Rose Wine	½ tsp
Curry Paste	2 tbsp
Satay Paste	1 tbsp

Sauce

Honey	2 tbsp
Tarragon Vitality™	a touch
Orange Vitality™	1 drop

Method

1. With some oil sauté the shallots, garlic, head of Chinese celery and fermented black bean until fragrant. Dish up and let cool. Add sugar, salt and the beaten egg to the ingredients. Mix well and put in a non reactive container, let it sit at room temperature overnight. This is the marinade.

2. When ready to roast the spare ribs, brush the Chinese rose wine onto the ribs. Pour marinade over the ribs and let it marinade for 30 minutes.

3. Preheat oven to 220F.

4. Drip off excess marinade from the spareribs. Roast in oven for 15 minutes. Take the spareribs out from the oven. Adjust oven to 240F. Flip the spareribs over and roast for another 15 minutes.

5. Brush honey mixture over the spareribs and roast for 5 minutes or until skin turns golden brown.

6. Brush with more mixture to finish.

True love is when you are willing to share your noodles

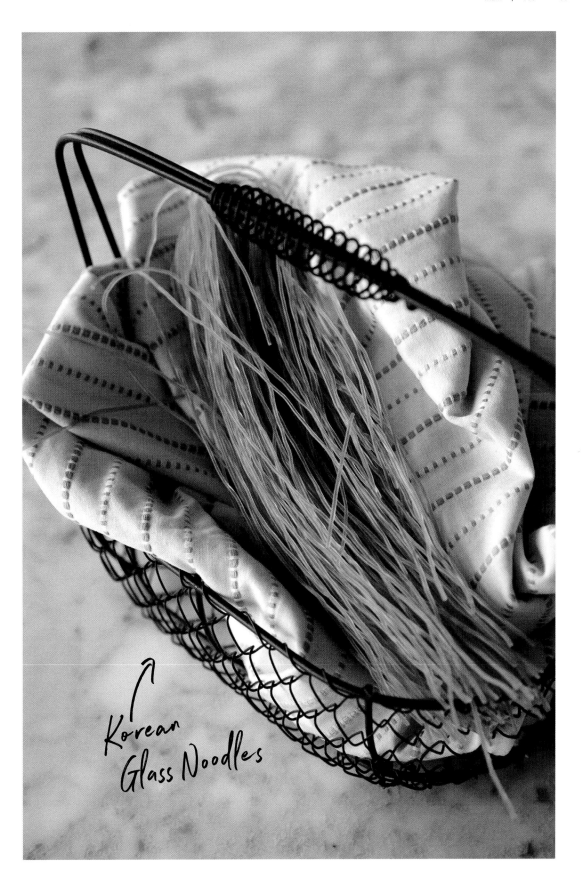

Korean
Glass Noodles

Clams Stir Fry in Rosemary Black Bean Sauce

This is a great supper standby. If you prepare the sauce ahead of time, this dish takes just minutes to put together. It makes a healthy and hearty dish too.

Try improvising and soon you will be making a new version of pasta vongole that will certainly impress your guests.

Ingredients

Clams	2lbs
Rosemary Black Bean Sauce (p.038)	1 portion
Ginger	3 slices
Garlic, sliced	3 cloves
Onion, sliced	¼
Chili	3
Sugar	1 tbsp
Arrowroot Flour	1 tbsp
Chicken Stock	½ cup
Cooking Oil	2 tbsp
Cooking wine	1 tbsp
Korean Glass Noodles	handful

(Soaked in hot water and drained; set aside.)

Tips

* Soaking the glass noodles in very hot water actually gets them to cooked. So when you add them to the sauce in the wok, you can finish the cooking more quickly.

Method

1. Soak the glass noodles in very hot water. You can leave them in the hot water until ready to add to the pan. (Before you add the noodles to the pan, drain them.)

2. Take the clams out from the freezer 20 minutes prior to cooking and put in a colander to defrost. Rinse and drain the excess water.

3. In a hot wok, heat the cooking oil. Stir fry ginger and onion until fragrant. Add in the garlic and chilli, take care not to burn them.

4. Add the clams to the wok and continue to stir fry. Cover for 1-2 minutes, checking once in between to see if they're opening. Once they start to open, remove the lid.

5. Quickly add in the cooking wine along the rim of the wok, followed by the Rosemary Black Bean Sauce. Toss well.

6. In a separate bowl, mix together the chicken stock and arrowroot flour. Add this to the wok along the rim and stir fry more until the sauce thickens. This should take 30 seconds.

7. Set clams aside leaving most of the sauce in the wok.

8. Place noodles into the wok and toss well in the sauce. Once the noodle is cooked, plate it on your serving plate. Pour the entire serving of clams over the noodles.

9. Serve with more chili and spring onion.

Rosemary Vitality

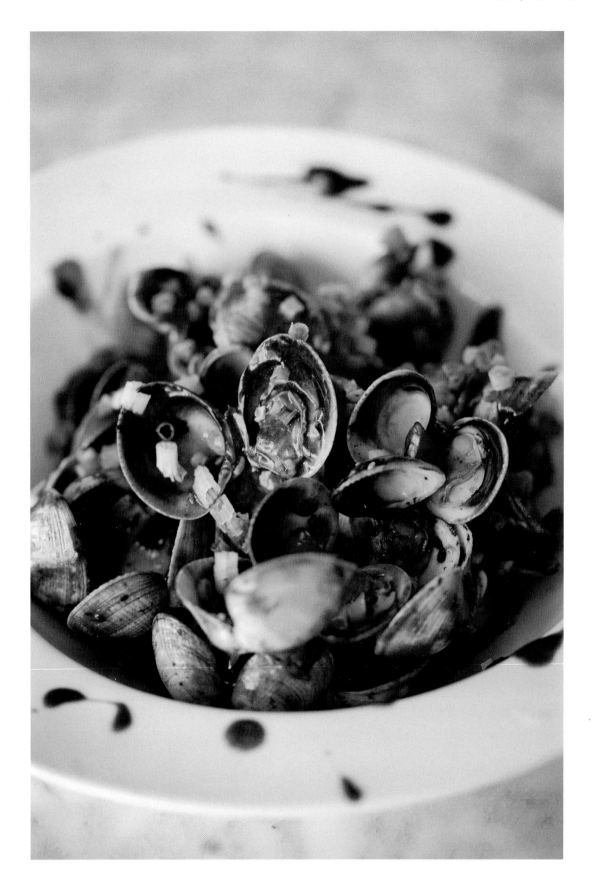

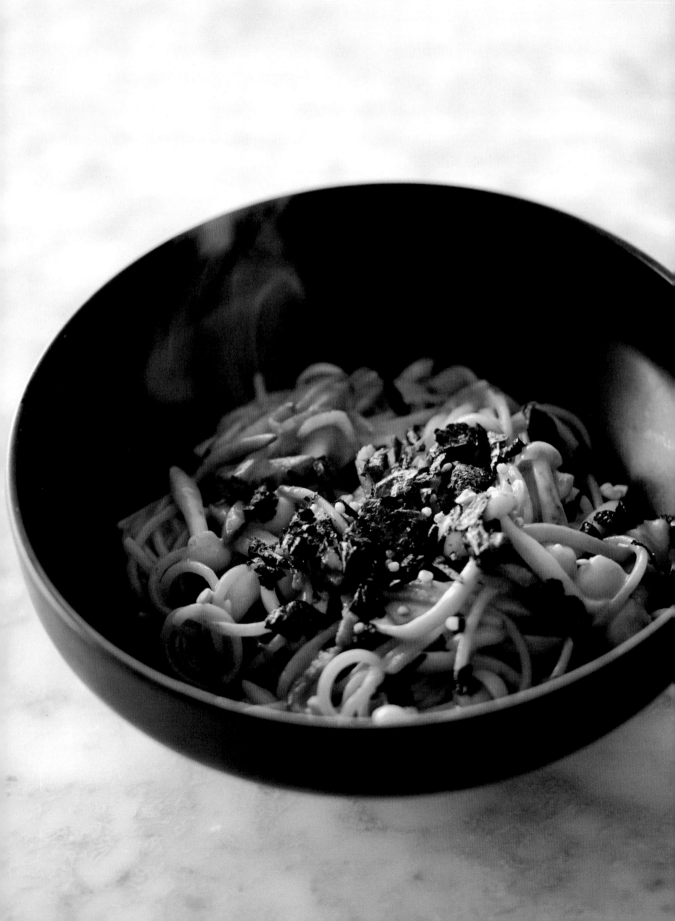

Lemon Jade
Shimeji Mushroom Pasta

Knowing how to cook doesn't mean you need to cook fancy. Sometimes the best meals are the ones cooked at home in the most simplistic ways. Just remember to season it with LOVE.

Ingredients

Spaghetti	4 oz
(I use True Grit Einkorn Young Living)	
A mix of Shimeji Mushrooms, Shitake Mushroom	4 oz
Cream / Coconut Cream	4 tbsp
Bacon, diced	2 oz
Soy Jade Lemon Butter Sauce (p.038)	4 tbsp
Seaweed Flakes / Furikake	sprinkle

Method

1. Cook spaghetti according to the instructions on the package. (I cook mine 9 minutes in a pot of boiling water and finish cooking them in the pan for an additional 2 minutes)

2. Meanwhile, sauté bacon and render its fat. Add mushrooms to the pan and continue to sauté until the mushrooms are cooked.

3. Add spaghetti to the pan together with the bacon and mushrooms finish cooking the pasta in the pan, adding a couple tablespoons of pasta water to the pan. Add in the soy jade lemon butter sauce. Toss well.

4. Add the cream if using.

5. To serve, top with seaweed flakes.

Jade
Lemon
Vitality

Chinese Recipe p.130

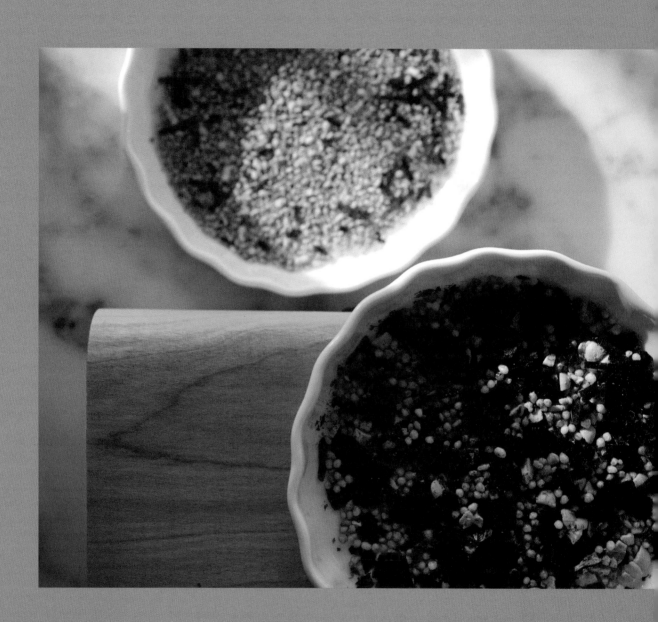

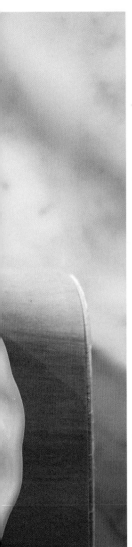
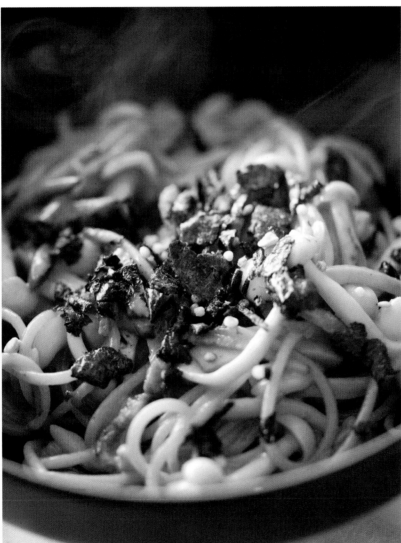

Spaghetti in Citrus Fresh Gojujang Sauce

This makes a flavorful pasta dish without having to use meat. The Citrus Fresh Gojujang Sauce is spicy and that's why it's important to use the egg yolk and seaweed to balance the flavor. The garlic flakes really give this dish a kick. Though it takes a little bit of skill to master not burning them (or they will taste bitter), it's totally worth it.

Ingredients

Spaghetti	4 oz
Seaweed	sprinkle
Sesame seeds	sprinkle
Enoki Mushrooms	3 oz
Fresh Egg	1
Olive Oil	2 tbsp
Garlic, thinly sliced	2 cloves
Citrus Fresh Gojujang Sauce (p.035)	3-4 tbsp

Method

1. In a pot with boiling water, carefully lower an egg and cook it for 3 minutes. After 3 minutes, take the egg out and run it under cold water to stop the cooking; then set aside.

2. Cook spaghetti according to instructions on the package. (I cook mine 9 minutes and finish the cooking in the pan with the sauce.)

3. Meanwhile, in a pan, with very low heat, put garlic slices into the pan one by one. Make sure they're not over lapping nor crowded together. You only want them golden, not browned; flipping once and take them out; put them on kitchen paper to soak up the excess oil.

4. The oil is now infused with the fragrance from the garlic. Sauté the enoki mushrooms in medium heat, adding more olive oil if needed (about 2-3 minutes).

5. The spaghetti should now be cooked for about 5 minutes now. With the help of tongs, take the spaghetti out from the pot and place them in the pan where the mushrooms are. Add a couple tablespoons of pasta water into the pan.

6. Add in the Citrus Fresh Gojujang Sauce and finish cooking the spaghetti in the pan. Tossing it so it is well coated with the sauce.

7. Transfer spaghetti onto a serving plate.

8. Crack the soft boiled egg and take only the yolk. Put the yolk on the top. Sprinkle with seaweed and sesame seeds.

Citrus Fresh Vitality

Chinese Recipe p.130

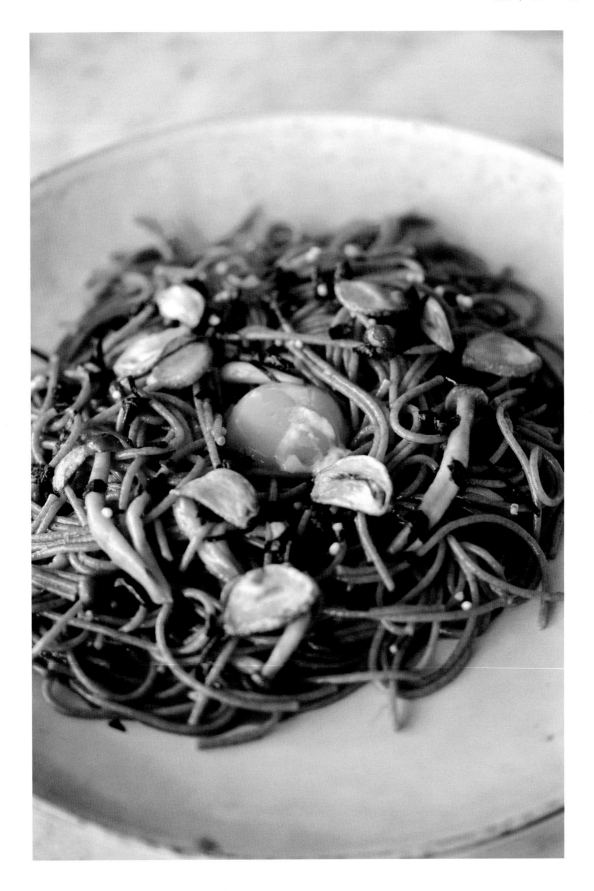

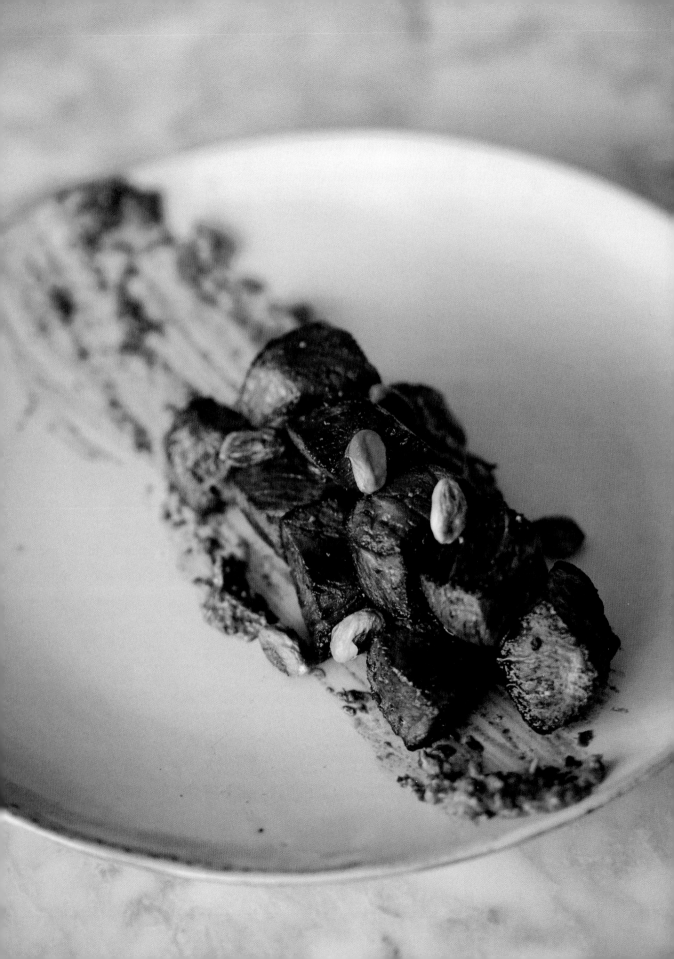

Stir Fry Beef Cubes with Basil Spinach Pesto Butter

Pesto is always beautiful in color and bursting with fresh herby flavor. With the help of Basil Vitality™, the flavor is simply exceptional. Remember pesto is always made to taste. Based on the ingredients, practice and play with your senses and adjust to your palette.

Ingredients

Ribeye Steak of about ¾" thick   total about 1 lb
(I use grassfed beef)

Garlic, minced   3 cloves
Cooking Oil   2 tbsp
Black Pepper   sprinkle

Seasoning

Soy sauce/ Tamari   1½ tbsp
Agave   1 tsp
Fish sauce   ½ tbsp

Sauce

Basil Spinach Pesto (p.034)   4 tbsp

Method

1. Cut steak into ¾" cubes.

2. Heat wok, and swirl in the cooking oil. When it is smoking hot, add the beef to stir fry. If your wok is not big enough, do this in separate batches. It is important that the heat is strong enough so the beef gets cooked quickly. If you see juices on the bottom of the wok, that means your wok is not hot enough. Either turn up the heat or reduce the amount of beef you stir fry per batch.

3. Add in the seasoning and stir to mix well.

4. To serve, spoon sauce on the bottom of a plate and plate beef on top.

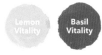

Chinese Recipe p.130

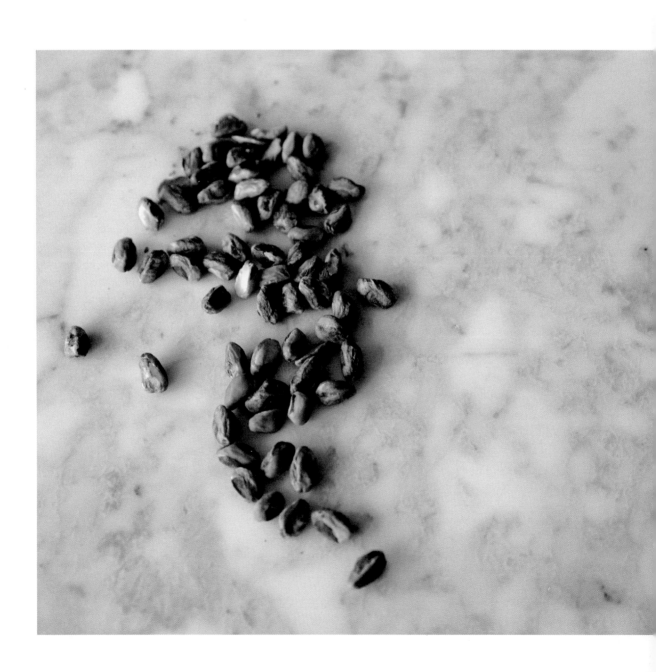

I totally regret eating healthy, said no-one ever.

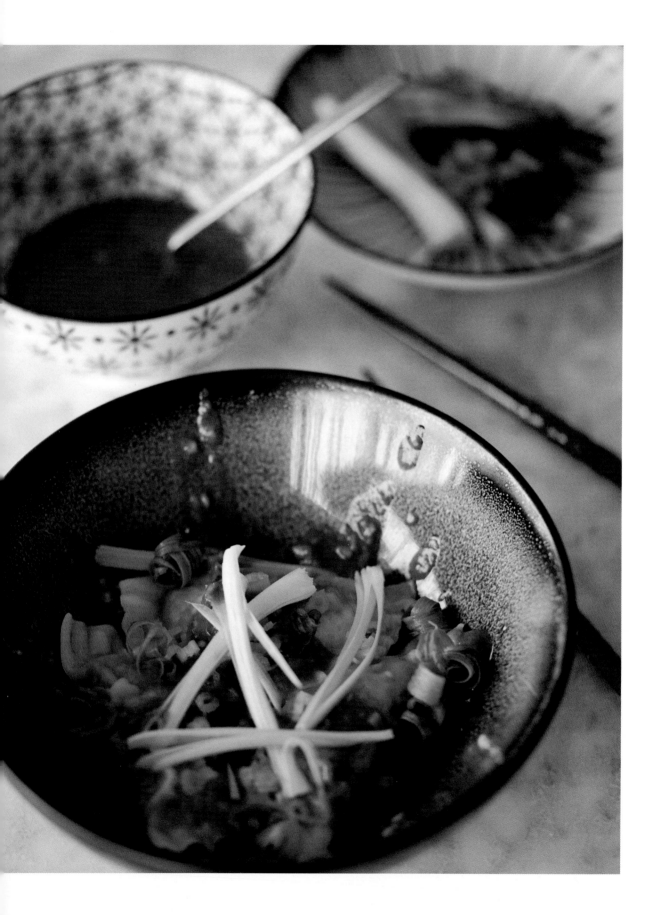

Wonton with Lemon Balsamic Tahini with Red Chili Oil

Dumpings are certainly a staple comfort food for many, especially in Asia. As little kids, my sister and I would be the little helpers, anxiously waiting by the side of the grown ups while they did the mincing and chopping. I can still smell the fresh aroma of the freshly chopped vegetables! I guess that's the magic of food and cooking; it brings back all those wonderful memories. Every time I have home made wontons, I can still sink my face into the steaming bowl of comfort, it warms my heart and nurtures my soul.

Ingredients

Wonton Wrappers	25

| For Stuffing |

Minced pork	4½ oz, with about ¼ fat
Spring Onion, finely chopped	8 stalks
Ginger, minced and juiced	1 ½"
Cooking wine	1 tsp
Tamari	2 tsp
Sugar	1 tsp
Lemon Balsamic Tahini with Red Chili Oil (p.037)	3 tbsp

Method

1. Put all ingredients for the stuffing in a large bowl. With the help of a spoon on a pair of chopsticks, mix ingredients clockwise for 20 times or until mixture becomes sticky.

2. Lay a wonton wrapper on your hand and put about1 ½ table tablespoons of stuffing in the middle. Fold the wrapper from bottom to top until they meet.

3. Fold the edges together and seal them together with a bit of water.

4. Repeat until you are finished with all wonton wrappers.

5. You can prepare this ahead of time until ready to serve. If you want to freeze them, put wonton on a floured plate, sprinkle more flour on top and put the entire plate into the freezer for about 30 minutes.

6. When hardened, take them out one by one and store them in a ziplock bag. These can be stored frozen for up to a month.

7. When ready to cook, boil a large pot of water to a boil.

8. Put dumplings in boiling water. When the water comes to a boil again, add a cup of cool water and continue to boil until the water comes to a full boil again. That's when the wonton is ready.

9. To plate, put a tablespoon of Lemon Balsamic Tahini sauce on the bottom of the bowl. Spoon wonton out from the pot and place in the bowl. Top with more sauce and chopped Chinese celery and spring onion.

Chinese Recipe p.131

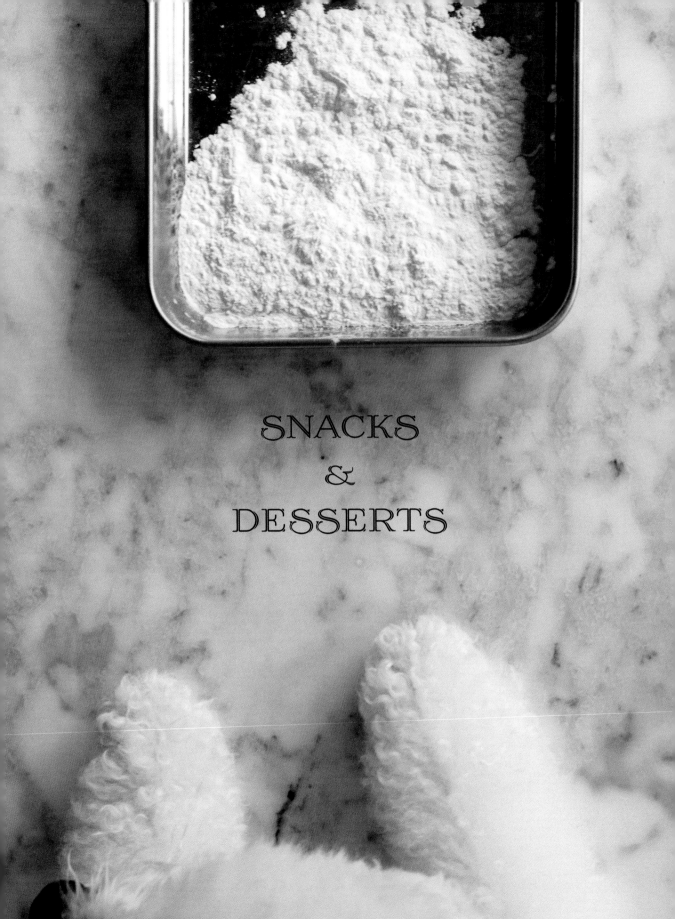

SNACKS
&
DESSERTS

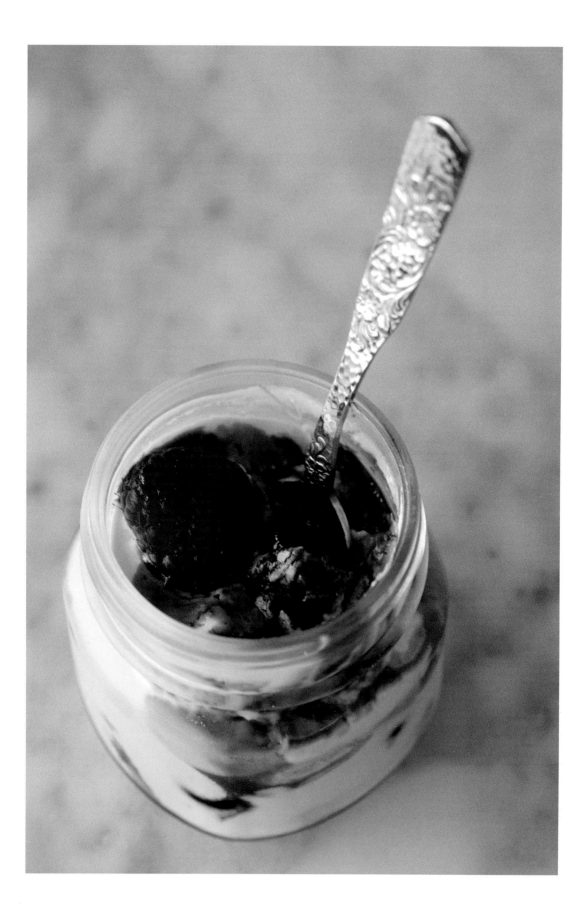

Berry Parfait with Orange Balsamic Glaze

This parfait is a cross between a parfait and a tiramisu. The tofu cream is light and is packed with protein. Almost guilt free except for the tiny bit of rum... so little it doesn't count.

Ingredients

Berries	4 ½ oz
Water	enough to cover the berries
Orange Vitality™	1 drop
Lady Fingers	9 pcs or Sponge Cake
Agave	2 tsp
Rum / Vodka	2 tbsp

| Tofu Cream |

Firm Tofu	10 oz
Maple Syrup	2-3 tbsp
Vanilla Extract	1 tsp

Orange Balsamic Glaze (p.035)	drizzle

Method

1. If using strawberries, trim off the stalks and prick holes on the them with a toothpick. For blueberries and raspberries, they're small enough to quickly soak up the alcohol, so there's no need to poke holes in them.

2. Put the berries in a sterilized jar.

3. Put a drop of Orange Vitality™ oil in the rum, and stir to mix well.

4. Pour the rum over the berries and into the jar; and top with filtered water. Store this in the fridge for 2 hours or up to 24 hours.

5. When ready to assemble, scoop the berries from the jar and reserve the rum mixture.

6. Take 2 tablespoons of this rum mixture and 2 tsp of agave to the mixture, stir to combine. You can adjust the sweetness to your liking by adding in more agave.

7. When ready to assemble, set up a station like this: the alcohol mixture, the lady fingers, the bowl of berries, tofu cream, and a glass container of about 4" x 4" (or glasses).

8. Dip the lady fingers one by one into the reserved rum from step 5, and immediately transfer them into the serving container. Spoon some berries on top and finish with a layer of tofu cream. Repeat so you get another layer of lady fingers, berries and tofu cream.

9. Put in the refrigerator for at least an hour to let it set.

10. Top with a drizzle of Orange Balsamic before serving.

Orange Vitality

Chinese Recipe p.131

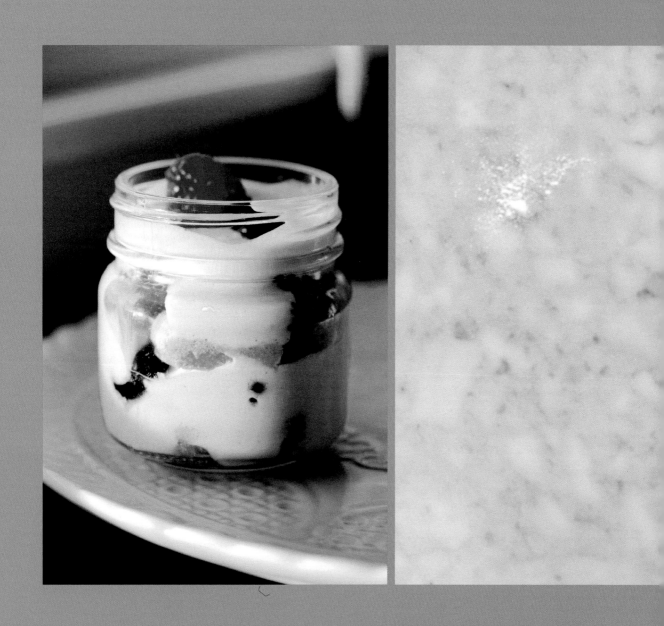

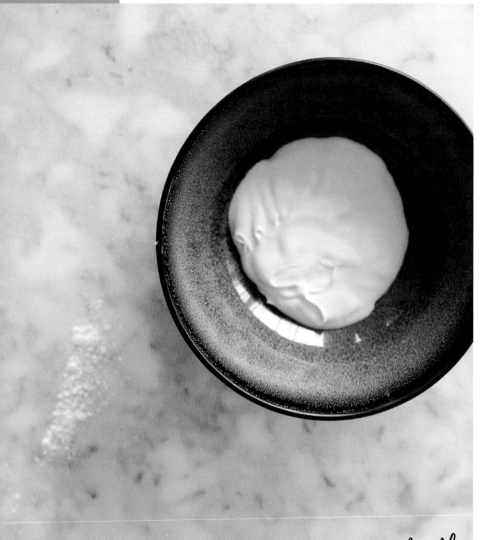

It is the sweet simple things in life which are the real ones after all.

Laura Ingalls Wilder

Dairy Free Cacao Peppermint Ice Cream

I can eat this all day. It's technically superfood right?

Ingredients

Coconut Cream	7 oz
Cacao Powder	4 tbsp
Maple Syrup	2 tbsp
(use grade B)	
Peppermint Vitality™	1 drop
Vanilla Extract	⅛ tsp
Salt	Pinch

Method

1. Combine all of the ingredients in a blender.

2. Blend until well incorporated.

3. Pour mixture into a freezer safe container.

4. Place in freezer for 6-8 hours, or until firm.

Tips

* If you cannot find coconut cream, use full fat coconut milk instead. Put canned coconut milk upside in the refrigerator the night before. When ready to use, open the can right side up and you'll find the coconut cream floating on top. Use the coconut cream and reserve the leftover liquid for other uses. Note that you'll need to use two cans of coconut milk in place of one can of coconut cream.

Peppermint Vitality

Chinese Recipe p.132 ➤

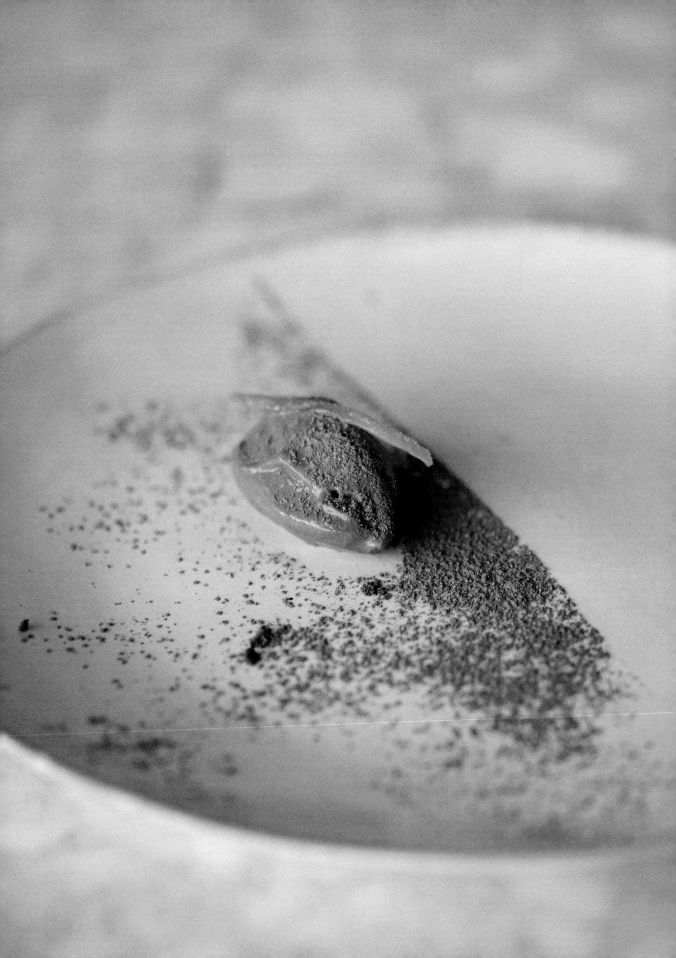

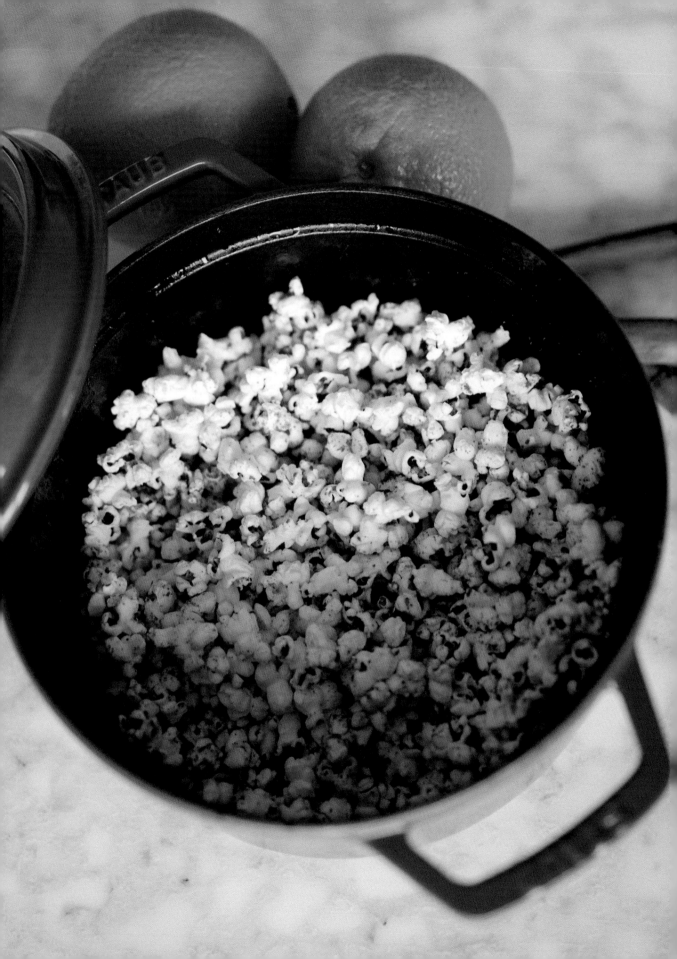

Cinnamon Tangerine Caramel Popcorn

Popcorn is so neutral in flavor, it can pretty much take up any flavor combination you can imagine... Try Lemon and Sage, Bergamot with a sprinkle of cacao powder, or an extra dollop of butter with black pepper. The combinations can be endless.

Ingredients

Oil	2 tbsp
Popcorn Kernels	⅓ cup
Butter or Ghee	1 tbsp
Tangerine Vitality™	2 drops
Cinnamon Bark Vitality™	1 drop
Almond Butter	2 tbsp
Maple Sugar / Coconut Sugar	3 tbsp
Vanilla Extract	1 ½ tsp

Method

1. Heat oil in a cast iron pot over medium heat. (I find using a cast iron cookware gives a much more even heat which results in perfect popped corn.)

2. When the oil is heated, throw in one or two popcorn kernels to test. When the oil is ready, the popcorn will pop! It's as easy as that.

3. Pour in all popcorn kernels and cover the lid.

4. Shake the pan to make sure all the kernels get popped.

5. When you hear there is no more of the popping sound, the popcorn is ready.

6. In a saucepan, put the ghee, almond butter, maple syrup or sugar, and vanilla extract and stir together over a medium heat until the mixture combines and turn into a thicker consistency or one that resembles a caramel. Then add Tangerine Vitality and Cinnamon Bark Vitality.

7. Drizzle the caramel over the popcorn and toss to coat the popcorn.

Chinese Recipe p.132

Lavender Taro Balls

This is a very soothing dessert; the taro balls are made with rice flour and tapioca starch, making them chewy in texture. By infusing chai tea to the coconut milk, it lightens the coconut flavor and brings the sweet soup to another level of sophistication. Adding Lavender Vitality to the taro balls makes this the ultimate comfort dessert.

Ingredients

Coconut Milk	9 ½ oz
Water	7 oz
Black Tea	2 teabags
(I use Chai)	
Lavender Vitality™	a hint
Taro	3 ½ oz
Tapioca Starch	1-2 oz
Rice Flour	2 ½ tsp
Coconut Sugar / Demerara Sugar	2 tsp
Lavender Vitality™	a touch
Water	(I use 3 tsp)

Method

1. Add coconut milk and water into a pot and bring to a simmer. Add tea bag and let it infuse for 30 minutes. With the back of a spoon, squeeze the teabags before taking them out. Discard the teabags.

2. Cut taro into small cubes and steam for 20 minutes or until cooked through.

3. When it's cooked through, take it out and place in a glass bowl. Add in the sugar and a drop of Lavender Vitality and mash down with a fork when it's still hot.

4. Add in the flour and start to knead it into a dough form. Adding water a little by little. (Each taro is different so there's no rule as to how much water to add in order to help the dough to form.)

5. The dough might feel a little crumbly but as long as you can bind it together, it is ok!

6. Form the dough into small balls of equal portions.

7. Bring the coconut milk to a boil and add in the taro balls to cook. When they float, they're ready to eat.

Lavender Vitality

Chinese Recipe p.132 ➜

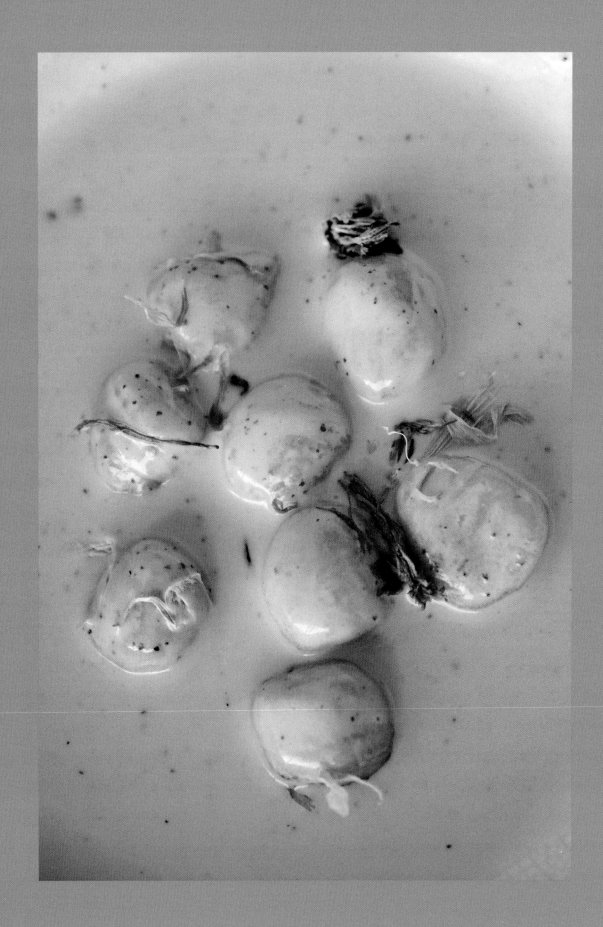

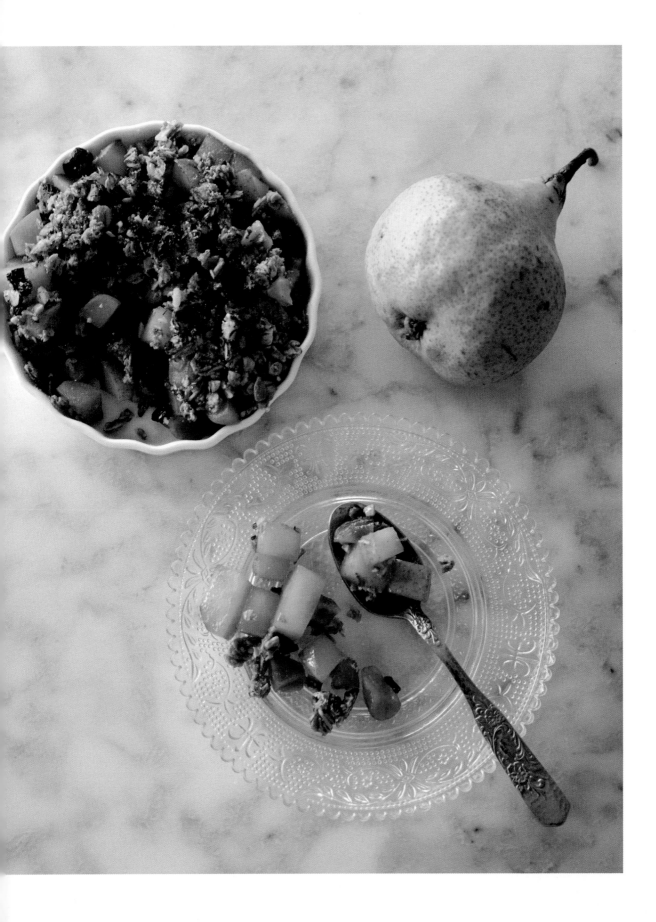

Pear Crumble Topped with Granola

Is this breakfast or is this dessert?

Sometimes all it takes is a different perspective when you look at things.

Ingredients

Butter	1 tbsp
Zest and Juice of Lemon	1
Water	2 ½ oz
Pears, peeled, cored and diced	2
Cranberries	⅓ cup
Apricots, diced	6
Coconut Sugar	2 tbsp
Vanilla Extract	½ tsp
Clove Vitality™	2 drops
Splash of Bourbon	(optional)
Salt	pinch
More Butter for topping the Granola	
Young Living Granola, crushed	about 1 cup

Method

1. In a pan, melt butter and sauté the pear, adding the lemon juice and the water. Continue to cook down the pear until softened.

2. Add in the rest of the ingredients. Cook for another 2 minutes.

3. Transfer the pear to an oven-proof dish that's large enough to hold all of the cooked pear.

4. Top pear mixture with crumbled granola and finish with dollops of butter on top.

5. Bake in preheated oven at 175C for 25 minutes.

Clove Vitality

Chinese Recipe p.133

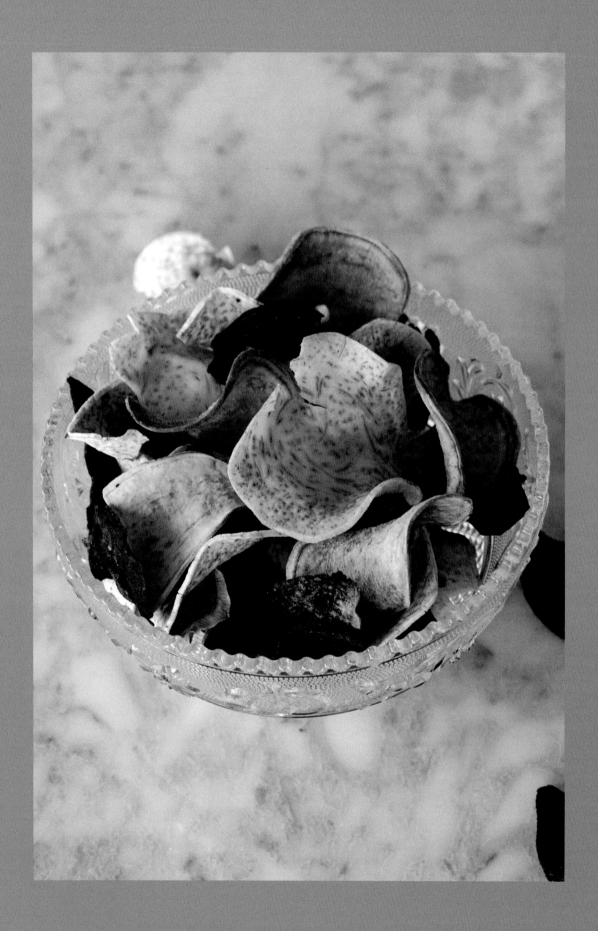

Root Chips with Rosemary Infused Olive Oil

Nom nom nom. These guilt free chips are too good to be true. Perfect for my down time sitting in front of the TV, and doing nothing.

Ingredients

Taro	3 oz
Sweet Purple Potato	3 oz
Sweet Yellow Potato	3 oz
Pure Virgin Olive Oil	enough to coat
Rosemary Vitality™	2-3 drops
Himalayan Salt	generous pinch

Method

1. Peel and cut taro and sweet potatoes into very thin slices. If using a mandolin, adjust to the thinnest setting.

2. In a separate bowl, mix olive oil with Rosemary Vitality and add in salt. For every 2 tbsp of olive oil, I add in 1 drop of Rosemary Vitality. As for the salt, be generous.

3. With the help of a brush, brush olive oil on both sides of the root slices. Place them on the rack of a dehydrator. Dehydrate at 145F for 8 hours.

4. If using an oven, set oven to 145F with fan on and slowly roast for 4 hours or until dry and crispy.

Rosemary Vitality

Chinese Recipe p.133

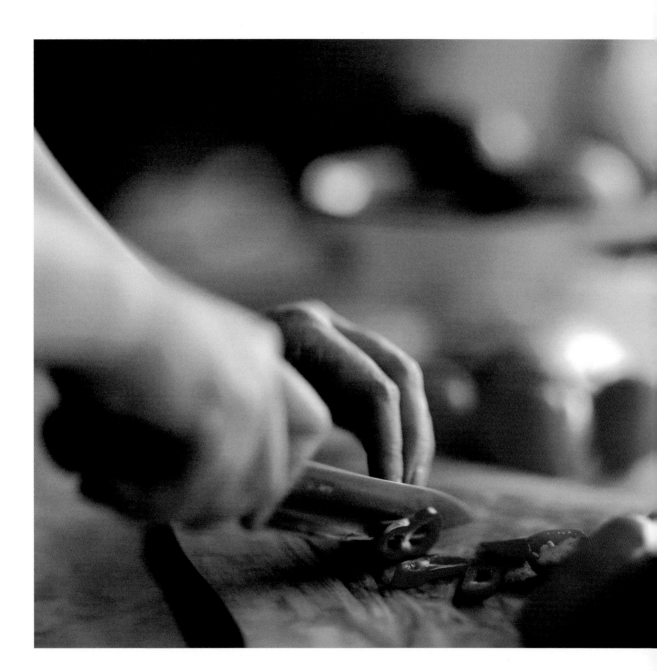

Do something today that
your future self
will thank you for.
Eat well, nurture yourself.

Xoxo Grace

醬汁

* 非常少量：用牙籤在樽口輕點一下

菠菜羅勒香草醬

當蘸醬汁，三文治，意粉，通心粉或烤肉都可以。

材料

烤核桃或松子	½ 杯
沙律菠菜葉	3 杯（100 克）
鯷魚	4 條（或用 Balacan 馬來西亞蝦醬 1 茶匙代替）
蒜頭	2 瓣
檸檬汁	1 湯匙
橄欖油	3 湯匙
檸檬精油調味料	1 滴
羅勒精油調味料	非常少量
鹽	½ 茶匙
龍舌蘭	½ 茶匙
新鮮黑胡椒碎	½ 茶匙

方法

1. 將菠菜，堅果，蒜頭，鯷魚 / 蝦醬，和檸檬汁放入攪拌機中。
2. 攪拌至粗粒。
3. 將橄欖油與檸檬油和羅勒油混合，然後加入攪拌器中。
4. 攪拌至混合均勻。
5. 用鹽和胡椒調味。

◗ 檸檬精油調味料   ● 羅勒精油調味料

黑胡椒醬

跟牛肉和雞肉都是絕配！

材料

乾蔥	8 個（或洋蔥 ½ 個，切碎）
蒜頭	4 瓣，切碎
牛油	1 湯匙
葛粉	2 湯匙
龍舌蘭	1 茶匙
糖	1 茶匙
高湯	400 毫升
老抽	½ 茶匙
蠔油	1 茶匙
黑胡椒精油調味料	4 滴
新鮮胡椒粉	¼ 茶匙
鹽	適量

方法

1. 在鍋中，用低溫把牛油融化；放入蒜粒和洋蔥粒，直到變成半透明的。 小心不要使用高溫，以免把它們燒焦。
2. 加入一茶匙新鮮胡椒粉，並炒香。
3. 加入葛粉，用勺子攪拌成麵糊。
4. 慢慢地把高湯倒入，並攪拌成醬。
5. 隨著醬汁變稠，加入龍舌蘭和鹽調味。
6. 關火，並添加黑胡椒精油調味料。

● 黑胡椒精油調味料

精油調配黑醋

與雞肉，鴨胸，番茄沙拉，草莓，冰淇淋相得益彰。

材料

黑醋	⅓ 杯
精油調味料（隨個人口味）	1 滴
龍舌蘭	1 茶匙
黑胡椒	適量（可選，若作甜品用，就要免去）
芝麻油	2 滴（可選，若作甜品用，就要免去）

方法

1. 在一個小鍋裡，慢火煮黑醋，直到份量減少至 ¼。需時約 6-7 分鐘（根據每款醋而定）。 請注意，當醋冷卻後，它會變稠。
2. 加入龍舌蘭，精油調味料、黑胡椒和芝麻油調味。

其他精油調味料建議：

● 甜橙精油調味料   ● 西柚精油調味料
● 薰衣草精油調味料   ● 佛手柑精油調味料

韓式柑橘辣醬

配海鮮和肉類都很好。 可以用作蘸醬，調味料或醃料。

材料

韓式辣醬	2 湯匙
Citrus Fresh 精油調味料	6 滴
龍舌蘭	2 湯匙
魚露	3 滴（建議紅船牌）
米醋	2 湯匙
橄欖油	1 湯匙
蒜頭	1 瓣，切碎
醬油	1 茶匙

方法

1. 將所有配料一起攪拌，直至混合均勻。

● Citrus Fresh 精油調味料

玉檸檬腐乳

配羊肉效果一流。可取替藍芝士汁作沙律醬用。

材料

腐乳	4 粒
玉檸檬精油調味料	2 滴
龍舌蘭	1 湯匙
芝麻油	4 滴
橄欖油	1 湯匙

方法

1. 在一個碗中，將腐乳粒與檸檬精油調味料混合在一起。
2. 加入龍舌蘭調味。
3. 加入芝麻油和橄欖油拌勻。

● 玉檸檬精油調味料

檸檬青檸辣醬

配鮑魚，蒸魚，烤豬頸肉都很出色。

材料

指天椒	1 隻
蒜頭	2 瓣
荷蘭芹	1 湯匙
檸檬精油調味料	1 滴
青檸精油調味料	1 滴
水	2 湯匙
魚露	2 湯匙
龍舌蘭	1 湯匙

方法

1. 將辣椒，蒜頭和荷蘭芹剁碎，放入瓶中。
2. 將其餘的配料加入瓶中搖勻。

○ 檸檬精油調味料 ● 青檸精油調味料

紅油檸檬黑醋芝麻醬

配冷面，青瓜沙律，雞肉沙律，餛飩都很好。

材料

辣椒油	1 湯匙
橄欖油	1 湯匙
蔥	1 茶匙
蒜頭	1 瓣，剁碎
黑醋	1 湯匙

醬油	¼ 茶匙
芝麻醬 / 花生醬	1 湯匙
龍舌蘭	1 茶匙
青檸精油調味料	3 滴

方法

充分攪拌直至均勻。

● 青檸精油調味料

花生蘸醬

材料

花生醬	1 湯匙
醬油	1 茶匙
龍舌蘭	1 茶匙
韓式柑橘辣醬（請參閱食譜 120 頁）	¼ 茶匙
青檸汁	半個

方法

充分攪拌直至均勻。

迷迭香豆豉醬

與麵類，麵條（Jajang Mien），蜆，青口都配合得很好。

材料

橄欖油	2 湯匙
中式豆豉醬	2 湯匙
迷迭香精油調味料	非常少量
生薑	1 片，切碎
蒜頭	1 瓣，切碎
蔥	切兩瓣
辣椒	1 隻
白胡椒	¼ 茶匙
龍舌蘭	1 茶匙
醬油	1 茶匙
魷魚墨汁	2 茶匙

方法

攪拌至均勻。

● 迷迭香精油調味料

玉檸檬牛油醬

這與海鮮和肉類都配搭得很好。

材料

牛油或酥油	1 湯匙
乾蔥	切薄片
蘋果醋	70 毫升
雞湯	3 湯匙
醬油	2 湯匙
味醂	1 湯匙
玉檸檬精油調味料	3 滴

方法

1. 在一個小鍋裡，把牛油加熱。 加入乾蔥片，炒香，注意不要炒焦。
2. 加入醋，雞湯和醬油；調小火。 直到份量減少一半。需時約 2-3 分鐘。
3. 關火，加入玉檸檬精油調味料。

● 玉檸檬精油調味料

百里香柑橘醬

配雞肉和蝦，美味提升！

材料

蒜頭	2 瓣，切碎
辣椒	2 隻，切碎（可選）
薑蓉	1 茶匙
柑橘精油調味料	3 滴
百里香精油調味料	1 滴
生薑精油調味料	適量
糖	1½ 湯匙
米醋	½ 湯匙
醬油	2 ½ 湯匙
芝麻油	2 茶匙

方法

1. 將所有材料（精油調味料除外）加到平底鍋中。
2. 使用低火力，將糖融化，並與其他材料攪拌成醬。
3. 關火，加入精油調味料。

● 柑橘精油調味料　　● 百里香精油調味料
● 生薑精油調味料

芥末柑橘莎莎醬

配烤魚和烤白肉，相得益彰。

材料

芥末醬	¾ 茶匙
橄欖油	2 ½ 盎司
荷蘭芹	⅓ 盎司
火箭菜	¼ 盎司
酸豆	2 湯匙（沖洗乾淨）
魚露	½ 湯匙
蒜頭	1 瓣，切碎
柑橘精油調味料	2 滴
檸檬精油調味料	2 滴
水	

方法

1. 把芥末放在一個小碗裡。 用手把橄欖油慢慢流入，用另一隻手攪動它。
2. 將芥末醬混合物放到攪拌機中，並將其餘成分加入其中。
3. 攪拌成醬泥狀。

● Citrus Fresh 精油調味料　　● 檸檬精油調味料

前菜

檸檬青檸辣汁鮑魚

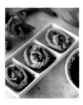

材料

罐頭鮑魚	1 罐（每罐約 12 隻）
冰糖	1 茶匙
黑芝麻	少量

醬汁

檸檬青檸辣汁	1 份

方法

1. 從罐頭中撈出鮑魚，倒掉汁液。
2. 把鮑魚轉到一個密封的玻璃瓶；將冰糖放進玻璃瓶。
3. 用蒸餾水把玻璃瓶填滿。確保鮑魚完全被水覆蓋。這有助清走罐頭汁液的鹹味。可於食用前數天先完成這步驟。
4. 從玻璃瓶裡取出鮑魚，底部（較硬的一面）界花，令鮑魚更易軟化及吸取醬汁。
5. 上盤時，把鮑魚放在盤子上，並在上面淋上檸檬青檸辣汁。

⚪ 檸檬精油調味料　　⚫ 青檸精油調味料

中華料理雜菌沙律

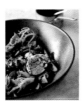

材料

半熟雞蛋	1 隻
木耳	1 盎司
鴻喜菇	1 盎司
冬菇	1 盎司，切粒
酥油	1 茶匙
健康豉油或豉油	1 茶匙
沙律雜菜	手抓份量
黑芝麻籽	½ 茶匙
蒜頭	1 瓣，切成薄片

特級冷壓橄欖油	2 湯匙
西柚黑醋	少量

方法

1. 先煮雞蛋。在小鍋中，放足以覆蓋雞蛋份量的水，煮沸。當水沸騰時，慢慢放入室溫雞蛋，煮沸 6 分鐘。拿出來，沖冷水。完全冷卻後，小心地剝下蛋殼。
2. 清洗沙律菜，瀝乾待用。
3. 在平底鍋裡，用低溫把橄欖油加熱。逐片的把蒜片平放在溫油中煎至開始稍變金黃。放在廚紙上把多餘的油份吸乾。
4. 將剛用來炸蒜片（已吸有蒜香味）的橄欖油倒入用來盛載沙律的大碗內，將其拌勻，以確保整個碗的內側被塗上一層油，把多餘的油倒掉，再將沙律菜放入碗中混合。
5. 在熱鍋中加入酥油，將所有的菇類炒 2-3 分鐘。用萬字醬油和黑胡椒調味。將木耳放在沙律菜上。
6. 把雞蛋切成兩半，放在沙律菜上。淋上西柚黑醋，撒上芝麻和蒜片。

⚫ 西柚精油調味料

烤獅子唐辛子伴玉檸檬腐乳

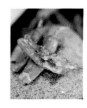

配料

獅子唐辛子	約 12 件
玉檸檬腐乳	1 湯匙
芝麻醬	1 湯匙

方法

1. 在已燒的熱平底鍋 / 鑄鐵平底鍋裡，把獅子唐辛子烤熟。當辣椒皮開始燒焦時，那就可以了。
2. 將腐乳和芝麻醬混合在一起。
3. 把腐亂麻醬混合物拌在獅子唐辛子上。
4. 撒上木魚碎裝飾。

⚪ 檸檬精油調味料　　⚫ 丁香精油調味料

羽衣甘藍脆片

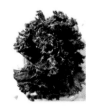

材料
羽衣甘藍	1 大束

醃料食譜 1
浸泡腰果	½ 杯
松子	¼ 杯子
檸檬精油調味料	8 滴
蒜頭	1 瓣,切碎
白味噌	2 湯匙
黑胡椒	半茶匙
紅皮藻	1 茶匙,切碎(可選)
橄欖油	2 湯匙
水	¼ 杯,用於細化
鹽	少量
辣椒醬	1 茶匙(可選)

醃料食譜 2
橄欖油	4 湯匙
蒜頭	1 瓣,切碎
檸檬精油調味料	3 滴
小茴香精油調味料	1 滴
鹽	適量
胡椒	適量

方法
1. 把醃料(橄欖油及紅皮藻除外)混合攪拌,最後才放橄欖油及紅皮藻,擱置待用。
2. 從羽衣甘藍上撕下葉片,按摩羽衣甘藍直至輕微軟化。
3. 把醃料加在羽衣甘藍上,輕力塗抹。
4. 在華氏 14 度下脫水 1.5 小時。

⚫ 玉檸檬精油調味料

主菜

芥末莎沙吞拿魚扒

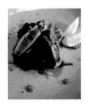

材料
吞拿魚扒	2 塊
菠菜葉	2 杯

吞拿魚醃料
橄欖油	1 湯匙
檸檬精油調味料	非常少量
蒜蓉	1 瓣
醬油 / 無黃豆豉油(Aminos)	1 湯匙
龍舌蘭	½ 湯匙
菠菜羅勒香草醬(請參閱食譜 120 頁)	3 湯匙

方法
1. 在鍋中放入 1 湯匙橄欖油,把菠菜葉炒至軟身。 加入鹽和胡椒調味。 擱置待用。
2. 在中熱的鍋中將吞拿魚扒的兩側烤焦。 每一面需約 1 分鐘左右。(按所需的烤熟程度,調整煎炸時間。)
3. 把菠菜放在碟子中間,並 將吞拿魚扒放在上面,然後在上面放上菠菜羅勒醬。 撒上黑芝麻裝飾。
4. 您也可將菠菜羅勒醬和橄欖油混合,製成醬汁點綴裝飾。

⚪ 檸檬精油調味料　　　⚫ 羅勒精油調味料

黑椒蕃茄燉牛肉

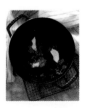

材料
牛肉	2 磅,厚切片(建議使用 USDA 草餵牛肉)
麵粉	3 湯匙
番茄	2 個,切塊
青椒	1 個,切薄片

蘑菇	1 包，切片
番茄醬	2 湯匙
辣椒粉	¼ 茶匙
牛肉高湯	¾ 杯子
酒	¼ 杯
芥末	2 茶匙
椰漿／酸奶油	5 盎司
醬油	½ 茶匙
鹽	少許
荷蘭芹	一束
油	2 湯匙
肉荳蔻精油調味料	2 滴

黑胡椒醬（請參閱食譜 120 頁）	1 份

方法

1. 先把砂鍋加熱，加一湯匙油。
2. 在牛肉中加上麵粉，然後加入砂鍋中，輕炒至變成棕色。擱置待用。
3. 在砂鍋中加入一湯匙油，放入青椒，炒至軟化。然後放蘑菇。把蔬菜擱置待用。
4. 將牛肉倒入砂鍋中，加入牛肉高湯，番茄醬，辣椒粉，芥末，醬油和肉荳蔻精油調味料。煮 25 分鐘。
5. 把青椒和蘑菇放回砂鍋，再煮 5 分鐘。
上盤時，加入酸奶油攪拌，並撒上荷蘭芹。

● 肉荳蔻油調味料　　　● 黑胡椒精油調味料

韓式柑橘辣醬炒豬肉

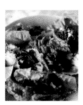

材料

梅頭豬肉	5 盎司，切成小條
蒜頭	1 瓣，切成片
生菜	4-5 塊
紫蘇葉／荷蘭芹	少量
蔥	2 棵
韓式鮮柑橘辣醬（請參閱食譜 120 頁）	4 湯匙
油	2 湯匙

方法

1. 將蔥切成兩部分。白色部分切成 2 寸長，把其餘部份切碎。
2. 在已加熱的鐵鍋裡，把油加熱。
3. 當油的溫度稍微提高時，將已切好的蒜頭放入鍋中，加熱至金黃色。然後將它們從鍋上取出，放在廚房紙巾上，以吸掉多餘的油份。
4. 在同一個鍋裡，放入蔥，炒至聞到香味。
5. 放入豬肉，翻炒。此時鍋正處於高溫狀態，豬肉會容易變焦。

當豬肉炒至七成熟時，加入半份韓式鮮柑橘辣醬，繼續翻炒。
6. 上盤時，先把生菜放在碟上，然後在生菜上放上紫蘇葉，再把豬肉放在上面。淋上更多辣醬和已切碎的蔥或荷蘭芹。

● Citrus Fresh 精油調味料

香辣黑醋脆雞翼

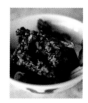

材料

雞中翼	10 隻
生薑精油調味料	3 滴
紹興酒	1 湯匙
雞蛋	1 隻
有機古老小麥粉	5 湯匙
蒜粉	1 茶匙
洋蔥粉	1 茶匙
精油黑醋醬汁（請參閱食譜 120 頁）	1 份
	（這食譜選用了西柚精油調味料）
生蜂蜜	1 湯匙
醬油或豉油	¼ 茶匙
辣椒油	¼ 茶匙
碎花生或芝麻	少量（裝飾用）

方法

1. 雞翼清洗乾淨及拍乾。垂直切開，每一塊只有一條骨。
2. 用生薑精油調味料和紹興酒把雞翼醃 15 分鐘。
3. 把雞翼取出，將多餘的醃汁倒掉。
4. 沾炸料：打蛋，並放在一個碗裡；在另一個碗或碟子中，將麵粉，蒜粉和洋蔥粉攪拌。先把雞翼浸在蛋汁內，然後把雞翼放在粉類混合物裡，把多餘的粉拍下。
5. 用中火，在熱油中炸約 2 分鐘，並確保在這之間把雞翼翻轉一次。取出雞翼。轉大火，再把雞翼煎 30-45 秒。把雞翼取出，放在廚房紙上，吸收多餘的油。
6. 同時，把西柚黑醋醬汁放在一個碗裡，與蜂蜜，醬油，辣椒油一起攪拌。
7. 把雞翼放在盛有醬汁的碗裡，與西柚黑醋汁拌勻。
8. 上盤時，在上面撒上紅辣椒片，芝麻或蔥。

● 生薑精油調味料　　　● 西柚精油調味料

左宗棠雞

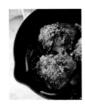

材料
雞腿肉	3 塊
葛粉 / 木薯粉	2 湯匙
食用油	1 湯匙
紅蔥頭	3 粒
蔥	2 條
芝麻	

醃料
紹興酒	1 湯匙
醬油 / 無黃豆豉油（Aminos）	1 茶匙
白胡椒粉	1/2 茶匙

醬料
百里香柑橘醬（請參閱食譜 122 頁）	1 份
雞高湯或水	3 湯匙

方法
1. 先將雞肉用醃料醃 15-20 分鐘。
2. 把多餘的醃料用廚房紙巾輕輕吸乾。
3. 在雞塊上平均撒上麵粉。可以輕輕拍打，把多餘的麵粉拍走。
4. 在已加熱的平底鍋裡放入食用油。
5. 先將蔥段和紅蔥頭爆香，後放到鍋邊。
6. 把雞腿放進鍋裡，雞皮部份朝下，在平底鍋煎約 6 分鐘，當表面變金黃色的時候翻轉，煮約 3 分鐘，或至雞肉不黏鍋。
7. 同時，將預先準備的醬汁和 3 湯匙水 / 高湯混合
8. 把醬汁加進鍋中，把鍋蓋上。轉慢火炆雞肉。（留意：醬汁只需要蓋至雞肉部份，雞皮部份可保留脆口）。
9. 用中火燉（煮）約 15 分鐘或至雞肉熟透。
10. 這時，醬汁應是濃稠且有光澤。若醬汁不夠濃稠，就把雞肉先取出放一旁，然後再加熱收汁，讓醬汁濃縮。
11. 上盤時，把醬汁淋在雞肉上，再在上面撒芝麻和蔥粒。

● 柑橘精油調味料　　● 百里香精油調味料
● 生薑精油調味料

日本芥末柑橘青醬烤鯖魚

材料
鯖魚	2 片
鹽	1 茶匙
橄欖油	½ 湯匙
芥末柑橘莎莎醬（請參閱食譜 122 頁）	½ 份

方法
1. 把鯖魚清洗乾淨，用廚房紙巾擦乾。
2. 在魚肉上撒上鹽。
3. 在魚皮上掃上橄欖油，再在魚皮上撒上更多的鹽。
4. 將鯖魚（魚皮朝上）放在已鋪上錫紙的烤盤上。
5. 焗爐預熱，然後把鯖魚用 180℃烤焗 10-15 分鐘，或直至魚皮有燒焦的顏色。
6. 上盤時，在烤好的鯖魚上放一勺日本芥茉柑橘青醬。如有需要，亦可淋上更多橄欖油。

上盤建議
* 簡單的羽衣甘藍沙律：只需把橄欖油，檸檬汁，鹽和蒜蓉混合成沙律汁，淋在羽衣甘藍上，並在上面撒上石榴和藜麥片。
* 從羽衣甘藍中挑出堅硬的莖，只留下菜葉。按摩菜葉，直到它們變軟。可以提前 2-3 小時把這沙律先準備好。

● Citrus Fresh 精油調味料　　● 檸檬精油調味料

玉檸檬雞翼

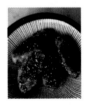

材料
雞中翼	8 隻
玉檸檬牛油醬（請參閱食譜 122 頁）	1 份
白芝麻（已炒）	2 湯匙
蔥（切碎）	1 湯匙
葛粉 / 木薯粉	4 湯匙
油	1 湯匙
蜂蜜	2 湯匙

方法
1. 先把雞翼清洗乾淨，並瀝乾。
2. 雞翼拍上葛粉 / 鷹粟粉，並用 1 湯匙熱油將它們煎至金黃色（雙面）。用筷子戳雞翼中間，以檢查他們煮熟與否。 若雞翼沒有血跡，那就代表它們已熟了。
3. 當雞翼在鍋裡煎煮的同時，把蜂蜜和芝麻攪入玉檸檬牛油醬內，拌勻待用。
4. 當雞翼完全熟透時，關火。倒入已混合的醬汁及蔥。 快速翻拌，讓雞翼沾滿醬汁便可以上碟。

● 玉檸檬精油調味料

玉檸檬燉羊腩

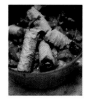

材料

威爾士羊腩	8 盎司
中式甜麵醬	3 湯匙
玉檸檬腐乳（請參閱食譜 121 頁）	1 份
馬蹄	6 顆（切成兩半）
白蘿蔔	1/2 個（切件）
腐竹	2 片
油	適量
紹興酒	1 湯匙
姜	2 片
老抽	2 茶匙
糖	½ 湯匙
葛粉	1 茶匙 + 1 湯匙水
水	

方法

1. 燒沸一鍋水，把羊腩飛水 10 分鐘。取出羊腩，水倒掉。
2. 將 1 湯匙油放入鍋中，油煮沸時，放入姜片。
3. 放入羊腩，把兩邊煎至金黃色。灑入紹興酒。
4. 倒入中式甜麵醬及翡翠檸檬豆醬，拌勻。
5. 放入馬蹄和水（水要把材料完全覆蓋）。燜 30 分鐘。
6. 加入白蘿蔔，腐竹，再煮 10 分鐘。
7. 將老抽及糖放入調味。
8. 在一個小碗中，將粟粉和 1 湯匙水拌勻成漿液。
9. 把粟粉漿加入鍋中，調大火至煮沸。同時，不斷攪拌，直到湯煮稠成汁的濃度。
10. 上碟時，把莞茜放在上面裝飾。

○ 玉檸檬精油調味料

墨西哥檸汁湯米粉

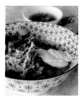

材料

| 豆腐醬 |

豆腐	4 盎司
橄欖油	1 茶匙
鹽	適量

| 湯麵 |

洋蔥	½ 個，切片
蒜頭	2 瓣，切碎
橄欖油	1 湯匙
雞胸肉	2 塊
雞湯	3 杯
羅馬蕃茄	4 個，切塊
牛至精油調味料	1 滴
檸檬青檸辣醬（請參閱食譜 121 頁）	3-4 湯匙
歐芹	小束，切碎
辣椒	1-2 顆（可選）
鹽	少許
米粉	2 份
新鮮青檸	1 個

方法

| 豆腐酸奶油 | （可以提前一天準備）

1. 將所有配料放入攪拌機，攪拌至奶油狀（約 1 分鐘）。
2. 冷藏不少於一個小時，以使其變稠。

| 湯麵 |

1. 在一個中熱的鍋中，用橄欖油把洋蔥和蒜蓉炒香。
2. 加入已切塊的蕃茄和雞湯，直至熳沸。
3. 在另一個鍋裡，把雞肉蒸熟，需時約 10-15 分鐘。
4. 當雞肉煮熟並且冷卻後，把雞肉撕出。
5. 把檸檬青檸辣醬加入沸騰的湯裡。把米粉放在湯裡煮約 8 分鐘。
6. 當麵條煮熟時，分成兩碗。把雞放在麵條上，並舀湯放入碗中。
7. 加入半個牛油果或一匙豆腐酸奶油，並在上

○ 檸檬精油調味料　　● 青檸精油調味料
● 牛至精油調味料

香茅酒釀帶子

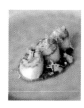

材料

帶子	6 粒（建議使用冷藏大尺寸魚生級別帶子）
椰漿	4 湯匙
雞肉	2 湯匙
龍舌蘭	½ 湯匙
酥油 / 牛油	1 顆
油	2 湯匙
菠蘿	4 顆，切塊
酒釀	1 份
檸檬香茅精油調味料	非常少量

方法

1. 將椰漿，龍舌蘭和雞肉加到酒釀裡。
2. 在鍋裡，把少許油加熱，把菠蘿炒約 10 秒，然後放在一邊。
3. 用高溫的油把牛油融化。當牛油融化時，將帶子的兩邊煎一下。您想雙面約成焦糖狀，但並不過熟。這將需約 1 分半鐘。擱置待用。
4. 在同一個鍋裡倒入酒釀混合物。這樣，混合物會從鍋裡吸收所有的精髓而變成棕色。
5. 上碟時，在碟上撒一匙醬。把帶子放在上面，用菠蘿塊伴碟。
6. 淋上橄欖油或用可食用的花卉裝飾。

● 檸檬香茅精油調味料

香茅番茄青口

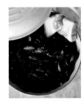

材料

| 番茄醬 |

羅馬番茄	14 盎司（建議選用連梗的細番茄，味道更鮮甜）
蒜頭	4 瓣
洋蔥粉	1 茶匙
蒜粉	1 茶匙
乾百里香	1 茶匙
鹽	適量
白葡萄酒 / 伏特加 / 酒 / 高湯	⅓ 杯
酒釀	1 湯匙
檸檬香茅精油調味料	非常少量
冷藏青口	1 磅
小麥意大利粉	少量（可選）

方法

1. 在烹飪 20 分鐘前，將冷藏青口從冰箱中取出解凍待用。
2. 將番茄，蒜瓣，洋蔥粉，蒜粉和百里香一起放入鍋中，煮沸。當配料煮沸後，加入酒或高湯。
3. 將火力調至最低，然後燉 30 分鐘。
4. 煨完後，把番茄皮取出。用鍋鏟將蒜瓣搗碎，放在鍋內。醬汁完成，可放在一旁待用。
5. 此時，冷藏青口應該已經解凍。把冰 / 水倒掉。
6. 青口放進中火的鍋中，然後加入 1 湯匙香茅酒釀。混合好。
7. 加入所有番茄醬，攪拌均勻。
8. 若這道菜做是做麵食的，你可依麵的長度折成兩半，放到鍋裡。
9. 把火關上，燉 8 分鐘。中間攪拌一次。
10. 趁熱時吃。

● 檸檬香茅精油調味料

辣椒雞

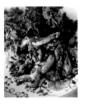

材料

雞腿 / 雞胸肉	1 磅，切片
油	⅓ 杯
姜	2 片
蒜頭	2 瓣
紅辣椒	3-4 隻，切大粒
羽衣甘藍脆片（請參閱食譜 124 頁）	

醃料（可選）

醬油	2 茶匙
紹興酒	1 湯匙

醬料

黑椒醬	4 湯匙
青胡椒 / 粉紅胡椒 / 四川胡椒	共 4 茶匙

方法

1. 鍋用中火加熱，加入 ⅓ 杯油。
2. 油溫到中等時，放入雞肉片炒至八成熟。移動雞肉，使它們不會粘在一起。此時，你並不想把雞肉炒至金黃色，相反，你只是在溫和慢慢地把它煮熟。
3. 把雞肉從鍋裡取出，擱置待用。
4. 只剩下 2 湯匙油，將其餘倒掉。
5. 放入姜，蒜頭和辣椒；煎香。注意不要燒焦。然後加入黑椒醬，胡椒粒；煎香。這步驟應該只需要幾秒鐘。
6. 加入雞肉，完成。
7. 上菜時，將雞肉放在盤子上，並用羽衣甘藍片裝

● 黑胡椒精油調味料

菠菜羅勒香烤羊架

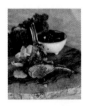

材料

羊架	1 件
芥末	2 湯匙（建議使用法國芥末，你也可以用第戎芥末）
菠菜羅勒香草醬（請參閱食譜 120 頁）	2 湯匙
菠菜羅勒香草醬（請參閱食譜 120 頁）	1 湯匙（上菜時用）
堅果牛奶 / 橄欖油	1 湯匙

方法

1. 將羊架從冰箱中取出。到室溫時，將羊架切成兩塊，每塊有 4 根肋骨。
2. 將芥末和羅勒菠菜香草醬攪拌在一起，將混合物塗 在羊架上。將羊架放在焗盤上，放置 10 分鐘。
3. 焗爐預熱至 230℃。放入羊架，焗 15 分鐘。將焗爐溫度降至 180℃，再焗 15 分鐘。
4. 用食物溫度計，檢查羊架的內部溫度。若是 60 C，那代表是三成熟；若是 68C，那代表是五成熟。
5. 當溫度達到要求時，從烤箱裡把羊架取出。用錫紙把烤架蓋上，讓它靜置 10 分鐘。
6. 同時，將等量的羅勒菠菜香草醬和堅果牛奶或橄欖油攪拌均勻。上菜時，淋在羊肉上。

上菜建議

* 羊肉配烤蒜，美味必然提升。
* 烤蒜：蒜頭從水平橫面切開成兩半，上面淋上橄欖油，用鹽調味，放入焗爐跟羊架一起烤焗。

⚪ 檸檬精油調味料　　　　⚫ 羅勒精油調味料

香橙龍蒿烤排骨

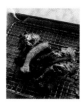

材料

豬肋骨	1 條（建議使用冷藏丹麥排骨）

醃料（需提前準備，需要不少於 8 小時發酵）

糖	4 湯匙
鹽	1/2 湯匙
蛋	1 隻
蔥	2 條
蒜頭	2 瓣
中式芹菜	1 莖
豆豉	1 湯匙（切碎）
中式玫瑰露酒	半茶匙
咖哩醬	2 湯匙
沙爹醬	1 湯匙

醬料

蜂蜜	2 湯匙
龍蒿	非常少量
甜橙精油調味料	1 滴

方法

1. 用油炒青蔥，大蒜，芹菜頭和豆豉，炒至香。滷汁：在已洗乾淨的碗內放入糖，鹽和雞蛋。充分混合並放入非反應性容器中，讓其在室溫下靜置過夜，待用。

2. 準備烤肋骨時，先將玫瑰露酒塗刷到豬肋骨上。把醃料倒在排骨上，醃 30 分鐘。
3. 將焗爐預熱至 220F。
4. 從排骨上倒掉多餘的醃汁。在焗爐中烤 15 分鐘。將排骨取出。焗爐調高至 240F。將排骨翻轉，再烤焗 15 分鐘。
5. 在排骨上刷蜂蜜混合物並烤 5 分鐘，直到變成金黃色。
6. 刷上更多的蜂蜜，完成。

⚪ 甜橙精油調味料　　　　⚫ 龍蒿精油調味料

迷迭香豆豉醬炒蜆

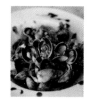

材料

蜆	2 磅（建議使用 WestHaven 可持續的冷藏蜆）
迷迭香豆豉醬（請參閱食譜 121 頁）	1 份
薑	3 片
蒜頭	3 瓣，切片
洋蔥	1/4 個，切片
辣椒	3 隻
糖	1 湯匙
葛粉 / 粟粉	1 湯匙
雞湯	1/2 杯
油	2 湯匙
煮食用酒	1 湯匙
韓式玻璃麵	手握份量，熱水浸泡後，瀝乾，擱置待用

方法

1. 將玻璃麵浸泡在熱水中。可把它們留在熱水中，直到準備烹煮。當你將麵條加入鍋中時，將水倒出。
2. 在烹飪 20 分鐘前，將蜆從冷箱取出，並放入篩中解凍並排出多餘水分。
3. 在熱鍋中把油加熱。炒香薑片和洋蔥。加入蒜片及辣椒，注意不要炒焦。
4. 將蜆放入鍋中繼續攪拌。覆上蓋 1-2 分鐘，檢查一次，看蜆是否已張開。若他們開始打開，取下蓋子。
5. 迅速在炒鍋邊緣加入料酒，然後加入迷迭香黑豆醬。炒勻。
6. 在另一個碗中，混合雞湯和粟粉。沿著鍋邊加入炒鍋中，再炒至醬汁變稠。這需時約 30 秒。
7. 把蜆放在一旁，大部分醬汁留在鍋裡。
8. 將麵條放入炒鍋中翻炒。麵條煮熟後，將其放在餐盤上。將全部蛤蜊倒入麵條中。
9. 上菜時，可配上更多的辣椒和蔥。

⚫ 迷迭香精油調味料

檸檬翡翠雜菌意粉

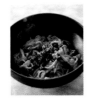

材料

意粉	4 盎司（建議使用 True Grit Einkorn Young Living）
鴻喜菇，香菇	4 盎司
奶油／椰漿	4 湯匙
煙肉	2 盎司，切粒
玉檸檬牛油醬（請參閱食譜 122 頁）	4 湯匙
紫菜片	適量

方法

1. 根據包裝上的說明烹調意粉。（我煮 9 分鐘，在鍋裡煮完最後 2 分鐘。）
2. 同時，把煙肉炒香。 將菇類放入鍋中繼續炒，直到菇類完全煮熟。
3. 把意粉加到鍋裡，並在鍋中繼續烹煮。加入數湯匙意大利面水，加入大豆玉檸檬牛油醬。 炒勻。
4. 加入奶油（如使用）。
5. 上菜時，放上紫菜片。

● 玉檸檬精油調味料

韓式柑橘辣醬意粉

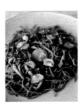

材料

意粉	4 盎司
紫菜	適量
芝麻籽	適量
金菇	3 盎司
新鮮雞蛋	1 隻
橄欖油	2 湯匙
蒜頭	2 瓣，切薄片
韓式柑橘辣醬（請參閱食譜 120 頁）	3-4 湯匙

方法

1. 在盛有開水的鍋中，小心地將雞蛋放下，並煮 3 分鐘。 3 分鐘後，將蛋取出並在冷水下運行以停止烹飪；擱置待用。
2. 根據包裝上的說明烹飪意大利麵條。（我煮 9 分鐘，然後用醬汁在鍋裡繼續烹煮）
3. 同時，在鍋內用很低的熱量，將蒜片逐一放入鍋中。確保他們不會交疊或擠在一起。你希望他們是金色的，而不是棕色；把蒜片翻轉一次，並將它們取出。放在廚房紙上，以吸收多餘的油。

4. 鍋裡的油現已帶有蒜香。用中火把金菇加熱，若有需要，可加入更多的橄欖油（約 2-3 分鐘）。
5. 意粉現在應該已經煮了 5 分鐘了。用鉗子從鍋中取出意粉，放入金菇所在的鍋內。並將幾湯匙意粉水加入鍋中。
6. 加入韓式柑橘辣醬，在鍋內烹飪意大利麵條。拋獲，以讓意粉更好的吸取醬汁。
7. 將意粉放到盤子上。
8. 打開雞蛋，只要蛋黃。把蛋黃放在麵上面。並撒上紫菜和芝麻。

● Citrus Fresh 精油調味料

香草醬炒牛肉粒

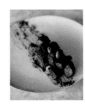

材料

肉眼牛扒	約 ¾" 厚，約 1 磅（建議用草食牛肉）
蒜頭	3 瓣，切碎
油	2 湯匙
黑胡椒	適量

調味料

醬油	1 ½ 湯匙
龍舌蘭	1 茶匙
魚露	1 ½ 湯匙

醬料

菠菜羅勒香草醬（請參閱食譜 120 頁）	4 湯匙

方法

1. 將牛扒切粒（每粒 ¾ 寸）。
2. 炒鍋加熱，放入油。 當油燒至高溫時，放入牛肉翻炒。 如果您的炒鍋不夠大，請分開數次翻炒。 注意，油溫高是很重要的！這樣牛肉才能快速煮熟。 如果你看到炒鍋底部有汁，那代表你的炒鍋不夠熱。 若是這樣，你便需要調高火力，或減少每次下鍋的牛肉份量。
3. 加入調味料，攪拌均勻。
4. 上菜時，先在碟上塗上一層醬料，其後在上面放牛肉粒。

● 檸檬精油調味料　　　● 羅勒精油調味料

紅油檸檬黑醋芝麻醬伴雲吞

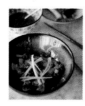

材料

雲吞皮	25 塊

餡料

豬肉	4 ½ 盎司，約 ¼ 脂肪
蔥	8 根莖，切碎
生薑	1 ½" 切碎和榨汁
酒	1 茶匙
醬油	2 茶匙
糖	1 茶匙
紅油檸檬黑醋芝麻醬（請參閱食譜 121 頁）	3 湯匙

方法

1. 將餡料中的所有材料放入大碗中，混合拌勻。
2. 在你手上放一塊雲吞皮，並在中間放入大約半湯匙餡料。從底部到頂部折疊包裝。
3. 將邊緣折疊在一起，並用少量水把它們黏在一起。
4. 重複步驟 2-3，直到完成包製所有雲吞。
5. 雲吞可預先包好，準備隨時烹煮。如果你想把它們冷藏，把雲吞放在一塊撒了麵粉的盤子上，然後在雲吞上面撒上更多麵粉，並把整個盤子放入冰箱約 30 分鐘。
6. 硬化後，將它們逐一取出，並存放在密實袋內，可冷藏一個月。
7. 準備烹煮時，將一大鍋水煮沸。
8. 把餃子放入沸水中。當水再次煮沸時，加入一杯冷水並繼續烹煮，直到水再次煮沸。這時，雲吞便完全熟透。
9. 上菜時，先在碗裡放一湯匙檸檬黑醋芝麻醬。從鍋裡勺出雲吞放在碗裡。再放上更多醬汁和已切碎的芹菜及蔥。

⬤ 青檸精油調味料

小食及甜品

香橙陳醋雜莓芭菲

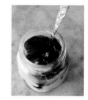

材料

雜莓	4 ½ 盎司
水	足以覆蓋漿果
甜橙精油調味料	1 滴
手指餅乾	9 件（或以海綿蛋糕代替）
龍舌蘭	2 茶匙
朗姆酒 / 伏特加	2 湯匙

豆腐奶油

硬豆腐	10 盎司
楓糖漿	2-3 湯匙
雲尼拿香精	1 茶匙
甜橙精油調配黑醋（請參閱食譜 120 頁）	撒滴

方法

1. 如果使用草莓，修剪莖稈，用牙籤在上面打孔。由於藍莓和覆盆子面積較小，可以快速吸收酒香，所以無需打孔。
2. 將雜莓放入已消毒的玻璃瓶中。
3. 將一滴甜橙精油調味料放入酒中，攪拌均勻。
4. 把伏特加倒在雜莓上，倒入罐子裡然後加水至雜莓完全覆蓋。將其存放在冰箱中 2-24 小時。
5. 準備上盤時，從罐子裡舀出漿果並保留酒汁。
6. 取 2 湯匙油，加 2 茶匙龍舌蘭，攪拌混合。（喜歡甜一點嗎？您可以加添多一點龍舌蘭！）
7. 是時候把所有材料合成了！先把材料依次整齊排列好：1. 手指餅 2. 橙油伏特加 3. 已加工的雜莓 4. 豆腐奶油，和玻璃容器（大概 4" X 4"）。
8. 將手指餅乾一個一個浸入酒中，又立即把它放到盛裝容器中。在上面鋪上一些雜莓，並塗上一層豆腐奶油。重複這步驟，以製成另一層手指餅乾，雜莓和豆腐奶油。
9. 置於冰箱至少一個小時。
10. 上桌前先撒滴香橙陳醋。

⬤ 甜橙精油調味料

薄荷可可冰淇林
（不含乳製品）

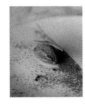

材料

椰漿	7 盎司
可可粉	4 湯匙
楓糖漿	2 湯匙（建議使用等級 B）
薄荷精油調味料	1 滴
雲尼拿香精	⅛ 茶匙
鹽	少許

方法

1. 把所有材料放入攪拌機混合。
2. 混合直到完全融入。
3. 將混合物倒入可冷藏的器皿中。
4. 放入冰箱 6-8 小時，或直至凝固。

備註

* 若沒有椰漿，可用全脂椰奶代替。 前一天晚上，先把椰奶罐頭上下倒轉放在冰箱裡。 需要使用時，才把罐頭倒回正確方向。打開罐子，用匙勺出浮在上面的奶油，剩餘的椰水可作其他用途。
* 請注意，您將需要使用兩罐椰奶以代替一罐椰子奶油的份量。

● 薄荷精油調味料

肉桂柑橘焦糖爆谷

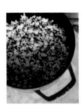

配料

油	2 湯匙
爆谷豆	⅓ 杯
牛油或酥油	1 湯匙
橘子精油調味料	2 滴
肉桂精油調味料	1 滴
杏仁牛油	2 湯匙
楓糖 / 椰糖	3 湯匙
雲呢拿油	1 ½ 茶匙

方法

1. 在中火的鑄鐵鍋中把油加熱。（使用鑄鐵炊具會熱量更均勻，有助烹調完美的爆谷。）
2. 當油加熱時，扔入一兩顆爆谷豆以測試熱力。當油準備好時，爆谷會爆開。就是如此的簡單！。

3. 此時，倒入所有爆谷豆，並把鍋蓋上。
4. 把鍋搖動以確保所有核都彈出。
5. 當你沒聽到更多的爆裂聲時，爆谷就準備好了。
6. 在平底鍋中，放入酥油，杏仁牛油，楓糖漿或糖和雲呢拿油，並在中溫下一起攪拌，直至混合物結合並變得稠密或類似焦糖的稠度。然後加入橘子精油調味料和肉桂精油調味料。
7. 把焦糖灑在爆谷上，然後拋爆谷以把焦糖塗上。

● 柑橘精油調味料　　　　● 桂皮精油調味料

薰衣草香芋球

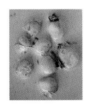

材料

椰奶	9 ½ 盎司
水	7 盎司
茶	2 茶包份量（建議用柴茶）
薰衣草精油調味料	
芋頭	3 ½ 盎司
木薯粉	1-2 盎司
米粉	2 ½ 茶匙
椰子糖 / 黑糖	2 茶匙
薰衣草精油調味料	非常少量
水	建議 3 茶匙

方法

1. 將椰奶及水倒入鍋中，慢火煮沸。關火後加入茶包，泡 30 分鐘。把茶包取出前先用勺子的背面輕壓茶包，然後把茶包取出丟棄。
2. 把芋頭切成小塊，蒸煮 20 分鐘或直至熟透。
3. 芋頭煮熟後，取出，放入玻璃碗中。加入糖和一滴薰衣草精油調味料，趁芋頭還熱時，用叉子搗碎。
4. 在芋頭泥中加入木薯粉、米粉，並揉成麵團狀。慢慢加水。（水的份量隨芋頭而訂，所以沒有規定添加多少水以幫助麵團形成。）
5. 麵團可能感覺有點脆，但只要你能把它們搓在一起就可以了。
6. 將麵團分成等份的小球。
7. 把椰奶煮沸，加入芋頭球煮熟。當他們浮起時，可以上盤了！

● 薰衣草油調味料

梨子金寶

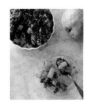

材料

牛油	1 湯匙
檸檬汁（連皮）	1 個
水	2 ½ 盎司
梨子	2 個（去皮，去核，切塊）
蔓越莓	⅓ 杯
杏桃	6 個，切粒
砂糖	2 湯匙
雲尼拿油	1/2 茶匙
丁香精油調味料	2 滴
波旁酒	數滴（可選）
鹽	少許
牛油	適量（用於頂層格蘭諾拉麥片）
Young Living 格蘭諾拉麥片	約 1 杯，切碎

方法

1. 在鍋裡把牛油融化，放入梨子炒，加入檸檬汁和水。 繼續把梨子煮熟，直到軟化。
2. 加入其餘材料。 再煮 2 分鐘。
3. 把梨子轉到一個足夠盛放所有梨子的焗盤中。
4. 在梨子上平均放上碎麥片，在麥片上放上牛油細粒 。
5. 在 175℃ 預熱的烤箱中焗 25 分鐘。

● 丁香精油調味料

迷迭香蔬菜片

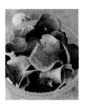

材料

芋頭	3 盎司
紫蕃薯	3 盎司
黃蕃薯	3 盎司
純橄欖油	適量
迷迭香精油調味料	2-3 滴
喜馬拉雅鹽	適量

方法

1. 把芋頭和蕃薯切成薄片。 如果使用 mandolin，把切片調到最薄的厚度。
2. 在另一個碗中，將橄欖油與迷迭香精油調味料混合，並加入

鹽。比例為每 2 湯匙橄欖油放入 1 滴迷迭香精油調味料。鹽的份量隨個人口味，可多放一點。

3. 使用油刷，在蔬菜片兩側刷上橄欖油。再把它們放在食物風乾機架上。 用 145℃脫水 8 小時。
4. 如果使用烤箱，請將烤箱的烤箱溫度設定為 145F，然後慢慢烤焗 4 小時，直至乾燥及香脆。

● 迷迭香精油調味料

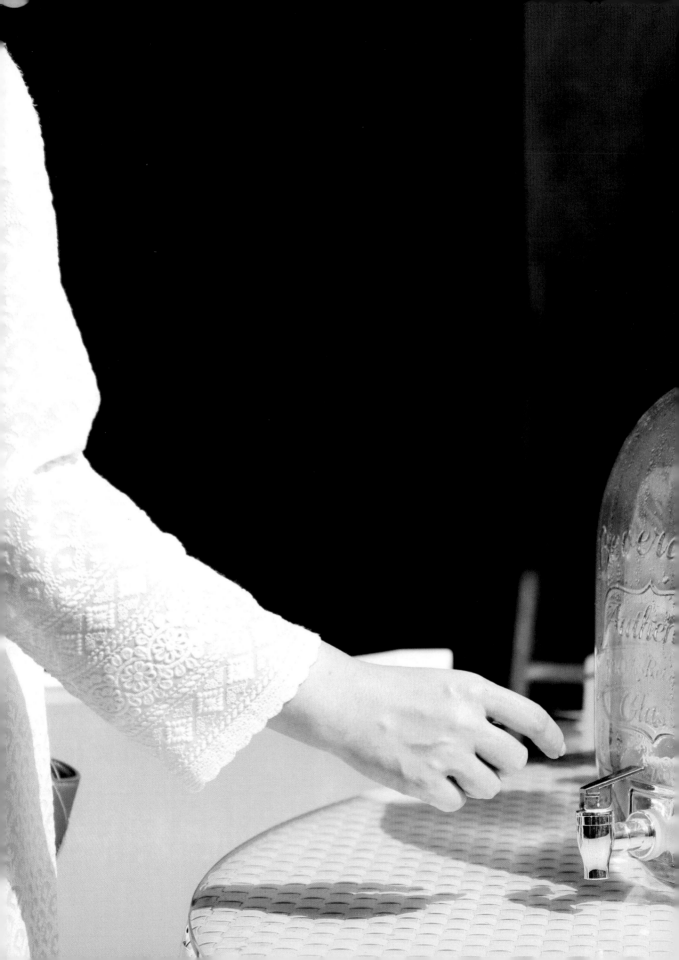